The International Library of Psychology

RELIGIOUS CONVERSION

T0174030

Founded by C. K. Ogden

The International Library of Psychology

PSYCHOLOGY AND RELIGION
In 6 Volumes

RELIGIOUS CONVERSION

A Bio-Psychological Study

SANTE DE SANCTIS

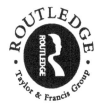

First published in 1927
by Routledge, Trench, Trubner & Co., Ltd.

Reprinted in 1999, 2000, 2001, 2002
by Routledge
2 Park Square, Milton Park, Abingdon, Oxfordshire OX14 4RN
711 Third Avenue, New York, NY 10017

First issued in paperback 2014
Routledge is an imprint of the Taylor and Francis Group, an informa company

Transferred to Digital Printing 2007

British Library Cataloguing in Publication Data
A CIP catalogue record for this book
is available from the British Library

Religious Conversion
ISBN 978-0-415-21111-6 (hpk)
ISBN 978-0-415-75815-4 (pbk)
Psychology and Religion: 6 Volumes
ISBN 978-0-415-21133-8
The International Library of Psychology: 204 Volumes
ISBN 978-0-415-19132-6

CONTENTS

PREFACE

I DEDICATE this book to my colleagues in medical psychiatry, in the belief that they, better than the psychologists by profession, will understand the disinterested and scientific attitude of the book.

This work is not intended for those who have the conception of psychology which has been usual in the past, and which is still often found to-day. The reader will find that it contains a psychology freed—as far as is possible—from arbitrary limitations. He will find it dealt with as an autonomous science with its own special aim (the reconstruction of the empirical Ego), and its own method (introspection)—though it avails itself also of the procedure common to the other sciences. He will find a psychology which employs only with particular reserve—I had almost written moderation, but that word seemed inadequate—both the philosophical method and the biological. He will find a psychology with a decided bent towards scientific objectivity, and distrustful of romantic subjectivity.

Such a psychology is, I readily admit, easily liable to misconception; not only by psychologists of certain schools and philosophers of almost all schools, but in particular by the medical alienists, who, just because they are mental pathologists, feel they are entirely justified in still reiterating purely philosophic maxims, in the ingenuous conviction that these constitute a modern psychological theory, at once bold and orthodox. It is strange that so many people should have apparently forgotten that philosophy—whether scientific, positive,

B

or natural—must inevitably remain philosophy and cannot be psychology. Indeed it is philosophy, at the present day, and not psychology, which, of all the contemporary sociological sciences, attempts the most audacious interpretations. Modern psychology, on the other hand, is far too much occupied to concern itself with such controversies as Free Will and Immanence. It no longer looks approvingly on excursions into other fields which it might once have regarded as heroic undertakings. In former days psychiatry was an amorphous hybrid. It appeared to be medicine, philosophy, sociology, anthropology, social hygiene, criminology, anatomy of the brain, morbid histology, and much else besides. In truth it was so indefinite as to be at once all and none of these things.

What modern psychologists would make of psychology is a science founded, not on inconclusive principles, but on working hypotheses, such as that of psychophysical parallelism ; a psychology assuredly poor, but unadorned and pure, and garbed neither as a slave nor as a sovereign.

I must avoid an easy misunderstanding. Philosophic thought there will certainly be in this very modest essay. Psychology, no more than any other of the natural sciences, can go out of its way to avoid it. We scientists employ philosophy whenever we establish the criterion of truth. Perhaps, after all, our working hypotheses are borrowed from philosophy. Even if it were possible to write of religious psychology without any reference to philosophy, this would not be in any sense commendable. But, on the other hand, no trace of philosophy which would obstruct the direct prosecution of the scientific method, or which would impede the untrammelled appreciation of phenomena is permissible to modern psychologists.

If a good many organic and biological phenomena are here introduced, the philosophical psychologists must not take fright. Without the aid of natural science, psychology is but a crude sketch, when it is not a mere pretentious unreality. It must never be forgotten that the man of science knows no psyche without life.

In discussing insanity and the neuroses, we warn the reader that psycho-pathology is merely applied psychology, and that it is neither histopathology nor philosophy. If we are concerned with conceptions apparently extraneous to science—like those of saintliness and religion—it implies that such conceptions are, in a certain aspect, also the material of psychology, as we shall see in the first chapter. Plato and the theologians are no longer the sole authorities on religion and holiness— the modern experimental psychologist may now discuss these questions without sinning in the direction of ' psychologism '.

This, however, by no means implies that it is the duty of psychology to find an explanation for all phenomena, nor, on the other hand, does it mean that certain fields of investigation shall in future be interdicted by definition. It would be well to state plainly that ' the sense of the mysterious ' is no longer to be regarded as in contradiction with positive science. Science does not admit of mystery, it is true, but this is applicable only to what science knows, and, given its methods, can know ; outside this field it has no opinions. This demarcation of the limitations of science has been expounded by Boutroux in his celebrated work, *Science et Religion dans la Philosophie contemporaine*. But even before its publication, William James had already swept away every objection which a sincere man of science could offer. Moreover, every scientist is in a position to give evidence. The sense of the infinite is not a virus which kills positive knowledge ; nor does the implicit recognition that there is a something which invests our spirit from without, undermine and corrode the intellect and make the student repent of having devoted the best years of his life to scientific research.

To such as would object that because of our caution we are deluding them or forcing them to work upon an ungrateful and fruitless soil, and who would reproach us for our failure to reach any definite conclusions, we must reply that psychology is unable to arrive at any conclusions, except in regard to its own objective. Since it lays claim to be a science, psychology, even though one of the least advanced, must logically be supposed to reach conclusions upon its subject only by such methods as obtain within the natural sciences.

After these prefatory remarks it will be evident why religious psychology must avoid, on the one hand, making itself the paladin of ' grace ', and on the other hand, of becoming the preceptor of unbelievers. The anxious reader, therefore, will search these pages vainly to find either the warm thrill of joy which faith gives or the chilly sneer of scepticism. Goethe, in his conversation with Eckermann on 6th June, 1831, making a brief comment on his recently completed poem, thus expressed himself upon the redemption of Faust : " This harmonizes perfectly with our conception of religion, according to which we save ourselves, not through our own strength alone, but through the strength of Divine Grace which is added to it." Goethe, in this statement, superseded all the psychology of his hero.

This book, however, modestly aims at describing the

processes of redemption outside of the works of ' grace '.
It endeavours to investigate the genesis, to establish the
relations, and, in the last instance, to indicate the data
for the recognition and the predictability of the occurrence
of religious phenomena in individuals immune from either
insanity or the neuropathic diseases. It will study the
appearance of these phenomena in persons who have not
displayed them for a long time, or who have never
consciously experienced religious emotions.

The attainment of so pretentious an aim is, as I realize,
not easy, since the theologians will insist on the inscrutable
prerogative of ' grace ', while the philosophers, on the
other hand, will defend the unpredictability of volitional
behaviour. In my concluding chapter I shall attempt to
reply to these contentions, without giving sure criteria
of predictability, but showing the possibility of eventually
establishing such criteria as soon as researches of positive
psychology, in a non-sectarian spirit, have elaborated
and refined our data.

With this premise, I have said what seems to me
necessary. I shall now offer the reader an explanation
of my personal reasons for writing this book.

The theme of the present work was not deliberately
chosen. It arose from incidental motives, though
powerful ones : a certain sympathy for the neglected
or maltreated arguments of men of science ; William
James's celebrated lectures on *Varieties of Religious
Experience* in 1905 ; the famous Congress of Religious
Psychologists at Geneva in 1909 ; the writings of
Professor Flournoy ; an interest in the stimulating
theories of Freud. The material was slowly but
constantly accumulated on my shelves, without any
idea of publication.

The first exhumation of my already voluminous notes occurred in 1918, when I decided—for no special reason—to devote a quarter of my university course to religious psychology. I happened at the same time to become acquainted with four converts to Catholicism, and my notes of their cases were used in my lectures, and now, together with others, in these pages.

These notes were again put away in my study, when a few months later, I responded to an invitation of the Italian Red Cross. There followed a lecture, of which I allowed an abstract to appear in *Bilychnis* and the daily press.

My preoccupation with the subject increased after this second exhumation. I read much, made notes upon notes, re-read whatever I had written on this and kindred themes; and the idea of the book took shape. The chapters began to grow during the summer vacation of 1921.

When the book was finally written, I began to ask myself if I were obeying some spiritual need in making a study of religion from a biological viewpoint. I had to explain why I had spent so much time in long and laborious reading, and in patient reflection, on a theme so restricted as conversion ; while I recognized how little I had added to the literature of the subject.

I came at length to suspect that my subconscious self had taken over the direction of my pen and my thoughts. I re-read the eight chapters of my manuscript to discover if my brain had been playing me some trick, but I still found the theme was not one which moved me especially.

Here it should be explained, however, that religion in general cannot fail to interest all who are capable of rising above the pitiful sordidness of daily existence. In these times of moral confusion, of hectic search for every form of physical enjoyment, of an arrivist and overweening science, it is only persons of callous spirit who cannot feel the enchantment of those regions of the soul in which goodness and idealism rule and inspire us to struggle against vileness and scepticism. There are moments, even long periods, when we thirst for something Ideal to raise us above all controversy, when we feel the need to close our eyes from the contemplation of brutality and injustice, and to take refuge in our innermost sanctuary. Whoever has not had such experiences can never feel the spirit of religion, or enjoy the poetry of goodness and the passion for life and humanity.

During the last half-century it is true that there has been a tendency for sociologists and positivist scientists not merely to under-estimate religion, but to dis-countenance all research connected with religious psychology. And yet that powerful thinker, Georges Sorel, although not a Catholic, has declared in the preface of his little book on the religion of to-day that : " If the true character of religion is so often badly misunderstood . . . it is because the sociologists have felt compelled almost completely to disfigure it . . . confounding it either with magic or with clerical abuses." To this statement I willingly add two positive facts. First, that at the present day it is demonstrable that the con-ception of God is *often* absent among uncivilized races, and, second, that it is *always* lacking—according to my own personal experiences as a psycho-pathologist—in idiots. To-day the conflict between science and religious faith is undoubtedly seen in a new light, materially different from the view of Taine, who saw it through the eyes of the eighteenth-century polemicists.

But in spite of all these convictions, I must confess

that so absurd an idea as to constitute myself the defender of morality and religion never entered my head. Besides, an entirely scientific research might not prove the best method of vindication.

So I was led to pose the opposite question. Could it be my subconscious aim to make a positive reaffirmation when all the time my conscious attitude was really agnostic? It would appear from Renda's deductions in *La Validità della Religione*—concerning which the reader is referred to the bibliographical notes to the first chapter —that he has no doubt whatever as to the unconscious bad faith of psychologists who deal with religion from the standpoint of agnosticism. Why, one might inquire of Renda, is agnosticism always a snare, when it can be prompted by valid general motives or the most impeccable personal ones? And cannot a psychologist, writing on religion, have no other philosophy than that of having none? Can he not place himself in the position of a critic or an investigator? Why can an agnostic neutrality never be credited to him? Must anyone who deals with religious arguments, if he is neither a philosopher nor a theologian, always be obliged to weary his readers with his personal Confessions? I shall allude to Renda's views again later. I merely mention them here as a point of personal interest.

But every attempt to plumb my unconscious was in vain. How often is the restless human mind incapable of comprehending itself. Consciousness exhausts itself in contradictions. Those individuals suffer keenly who, without being sceptics, oscillate between an unwelcome conviction that the reason cannot explain everything and an inability to believe by an act of will; who, whilst following the hard path of duty, disregard all those profound inner urgings which they consider irrational,

and turn towards science for the satisfaction of their
desires on a different plane. After re-examining all
possible motives, I decided that my true motive for
publication was that as a rule my scientific colleagues
of the laboratories and hospitals ignore religion. They
will continue to ignore it so long as it is defamed
in writing, in lectures, and in conversation, even though
it is still—traditionally—practised. This is an evil,
for there comes a moment in every life when the
questions will be asked: Can God be found by an
act of pure thought; or in the energy by which the
universe is moved; or in what transcends nature
and the human spirit? Why is it that faith, to all
appearances a thing so puerile, should in actuality be
so powerful? Is rational knowledge enough to live by?
What are we and whither are we going? Why do we
secretly feel that duty and love of our neighbour are
right? Here are questions that have been put to me by
colleagues in intimate conversations and in moments of
sincerity.

If all the arguments for and against religious psychology
discussed at Geneva were to be debated again to-day,
I think that its justification for biologists and psychologists would be found in this: that like the study of
history, religious psychology constitutes an excellent
preparation for the solution of the problem of religion.

The academic biologists view books which deal with
religion with suspicion, as my experience in university
circles has shown me. They even prefer the literature
of mediumism or of telepathy—because these possess
a more scientific air. My university experience, however,
also persuades me that by the side of the historical
study of religion which is once more in vogue to-day,

the study of religious psychology will be beneficial to all men of good will who, finding themselves confronted by the critical phases of religious thought, are seeking to discover light and certainty.

It has often been questioned whether—ethical considerations apart—it is better to cultivate all, or a few, of the regions of the soul. Who can tell? The pedagogues do not agree, but in any case it is better to become acquainted with these experiences, before cultivating or rejecting them. Whoever reads this book must forgive me if, instead of discovering the thinker or the artist, he sometimes finds in it the technician or the didactician. To those who smile sceptically at its foreword and who, therefore, do not read it, I owe no excuses.

SANTE DE SANCTIS

CHAPTER I

CONTEMPORARY RELIGIOUS PSYCHOLOGY : ITS SCOPE AND METHODS

IN dealing with any theme of a religious character we are faced at the outset by a serious problem ; the problem of excluding what is irrelevant.

Religion is something more than the object of psychological study. It is also the object of various other disciplines : theology, history, philosophy, anthropology, and sociology. The psychologist should clearly restrict himself to what concerns him. But it is by no means easy to determine the bounds of the psychologist's territory. It therefore seems appropriate for me, as a physician and a bio-psychologist, to determine the limits of my subject-matter.

It may be that by this limitation of the scope of my contribution to so contentious a subject I may secure the indulgence of my readers, for nothing is so calculated to rouse the opposition of those who would learn—or criticize—as the presumptions of a writer. The psychologist, however, must do more than enunciate his good intentions : he must frankly state the point at which he is aiming, and the field which he proposes to cover. The writer does not presume to create his own method in order to gain personal ends. He rather hopes to keep to the method of science and thus make a modest contribution to the ' science of religious experience '.

Before proceeding further it may be convenient, by way of introduction, to sketch in brief outline the methods of contemporary science which may be applied to the psychological study of mystic and religious phenomena.

Since Schleiermacher's demonstration of the possibility of a scientific analysis of the religious sentiment, and especially since the aims and technical methods of modern psychology have been clearly determined, there has been an ever-increasing number of psychologists who have occupied themselves with religious phenomena, with a point of view as different from that of the ethnologists and sociologists (positivist or otherwise) as it is from that of the apologists. There was, therefore, a perfectly clear tradition — Wundt, William James, Ribot, Flournoy, and Leuba—when the Sixth International Congress of Psychology, held at Geneva in 1909, took up the subject. It was thoroughly discussed at Geneva and—the extremists excepted—an agreement was finally reached.[1] From that time onwards *religious psychology*, as Professor Flournoy called it, had domiciliary rights in the framework of contemporary psychology.[2] The Jesuit, Father Pacheu, who attended the discussion, opposed the extremists, but did not actually object either to the conceptions or the method of the psychology of religion.[3] Another Jesuit present, Father Roupain, mistakenly subjected to hostile criticism [4] the psychological study of Gonzague Truc on the ' state of grace '.[5] To-day psychologists are all agreed with Höffding who declared that " the belief that a phenomenon loses its value when it is understood is nothing but a superstition or an immoral scepticism ".[6]

No one, at the present time, thinks that the philosopher, Adrian Sixte, in Paul Bourget's novel, *Le Disciple*, was justified in attempting to write a ' Psychology of God ' The Personal Deity of religion is beyond the province of psychology, and the search for Him in the substance or dynamics of our thoughts [7] does not lead to the truth ; Leuba's researches [8] failed to discover Him, and those Catholics who believed themselves to have been more successful must have been bitterly disillusioned by the Papal Encyclical *Pascendi*.[9] If God, the Transcendent, is to be found, it must be by other than empirical methods. Bacon, indeed, long since excluded the experimental method in regard to ' divine things '.

Professor Flournoy himself formulated the methods to be employed by scientific psychology in regard to religion. He laid down the two following guiding principles : first, the exclusion of the Transcendental and of any apologetic whatsoever of Immanence ; second, the biological interpretation of religious phenomena.[10]

The first of these principles has always been maintained by psychologists, including Ribot ; while the second is an incontestable postulate of contemporary psychology.

The procedure of religious psychology is therefore governed by these two generally admitted principles— (*a*) an agnosticism ; which is the saving postulate of scientific psychological research : and (*b*) the necessary connection of the phenomena of human psychology with vital phenomena ; this is the unassailable foundation of modern psychology, in opposition to the older schools of psychological opinion on the one hand, and to the *epigoni* of modern idealism on the other. Discussion of the latter of these two principles is now waning ; but psychological agnosticism, though accepted by many, still tends to be fervidly debated and cannot claim to have met with universal consent.

The exclusion of the transcendental implies the admission that every purely psychological explanation must be found within the subject and not outside; not, however, in a sense involving a philosophy of immanence. A certain kind of immanence is, of course, implicit in the positive or scientific method, which is essentially genetic. With such *immanentism* as this— if it may be so termed—scientific psychology cannot and does not desire to dispense; since to do so would be to limit the inquiry to a mere descriptive form of study—to a pure phenomonology; whereas it is our desire that religious psychology, like all the other sciences— such as physiology, for instance—may be explicative as well.[11]

Modern religious psychology, it is necessary to emphasize, in order to avoid misconceptions by the reader, is neither idealistic nor Kantian. Our attitude is certainly subjectivist, but within the limits of scientific psychology; whereas idealistic subjectivism is definitive in so far as it applies to the explanation of the Universe and of Spirit. For absolute idealism, the whole of religious life is confined within a closed circle; there can be no God outside of the Individual Spirit which is also the Universal Spirit. On this account it is to-day more necessary than ever to insist that the *psychology of religion* has to be kept distinct from the *philosophy of religion*. Their aims and methods are different, and the latter can treat of questions with which the former has no concern.[12] We would even go further and state that we here intend to disregard such problems as to whether the psychology of religion actually forms part of the philosophy of religion, which is Höffding's opinion, because we do not wish to change the nature of a scientific investigation by any preliminary compromise.

It is, however, to be hoped that these conceptions will not fall under the criticism which Benedetto Croce levelled many years ago against the empirical method in philosophy; [13] first, because the criticism of this eminent thinker was concerned with philosophers who wished to think as empiricists; and further for the very much more substantial reason that for him the empirical must be purely empirical, which is precisely what we ourselves believe. Croce, however, denies all possibility of an empirical psychology; and therefore has little encouragement to offer us in the task which we have undertaken.

The science of psychology has in future to avoid ambiguity, and in the interests of lucidity it is forced to disentangle itself from philosophic speculations, both as regards its methods and its aims. We propose here to hold fast to experience. Every psychologist knows that converts are unanimous in declaring that they feel before them the Great Objective; an external force, or ' grace ', or God, works within them for their salvation; and that to which they turn and towards which they aspire, is for them a living reality. They both implicitly and explicitly reaffirm the Judaic Hellenic Christian dualism. This phenomenon, so luminous in the consciousness of the religious soul, is capable of various explanations, by the dualist or the positivist, the idealist or the occultist. But for the psychologist it is an empirical fact, not amenable to discussion.

It may even be that the believer projects his states of soul outside himself, as in a mirror, so that he incarnates himself in the supernatural, creating for himself his own God and his own Heaven, as Gentile believes.[14] This is the idealistic dogma, which is all very well; but the fact remains that the believer actually lives in the sight of God and in His Kingdom and that this reality informs his mind and his spirit.

It would, for every reason, be futile to attempt to draw from our empirical realism conclusions savouring of apologetics. It has been suggested by some that religious psychology should proceed by the application of John Stuart Mill's Method of Residues, one of the experimental methods which that philosopher derived from Bacon. But Höffding, who rightly disagrees on this point with Bertrand, considers that, according to this method, the 'residuum' for the man of science is not God, but the Unknown.[15] For the rest it is clear that Father Pacheu could not have thought otherwise, if we recall that, according to him, scientific psychology "ignores the first and superior cause; and religious psychology may be undertaken by any Catholic whatsoever; much more so since Catholicism is not based upon the ecstasy of St. Theresa". His admonition should be taken to heart by many fanatics, who would also be well advised to peruse the works of Benedict XIV.

Father Thomas Mainage[16] was distressed by the Protestant writer Berguer,[17] because the latter detected transcendentalism in his *Psychologie de la Conversion*; and retorted with the claim that Berguer had "*l'esprit paralysé par des ' options' metaphysiques*", and, in particular '*d'options Kantiennes*'. It is a fact, however, that Mainage admitted that he did not exclude transcendentalism from his psychology; and that he is therefore in error—according to the view of contemporary psychology—is evident.

It is strange that Alfred Renda[18] should have wished to reopen the debate in his recent work on religious dialectics. Renda is thoroughly sceptical as to 'psychological neutrality'. He regards the study of religious psychology as an "unsuspected ambush . . . the most seductive, the most ingenious, the subtlest conceivable means for blocking the way of speculation in the territory into which it makes friendly but devastating incursions". This attitude is, however, either a gratuitous insult to the science, or an ingenuous and confused identification of it with some prejudiced psychologist. On the other hand, it is very difficult to believe these criticisms justified in individual instances. It may suffice here to point to Professor Flournoy, the original advocate of the ' neutrality' of religious psychology, who was not only a great and good man, but was also a religious soul like William James ; while Leuba, to whom we owe so many psychological studies on religion, has never concealed his own austere positivism.

In reality modern psychology makes no claim to exhaust religion with its researches, nor does it regard the residue that it leaves as the stubble left after the mowing. The reason for agnosticism is implicit in the objectives and methods of contemporary psychology. In dealing with religious psychology, then, the attitude of agnostic neutrality becomes doubly necessary. It is a necessary concomitant of the present phase of development which has now been reached by this new branch of applied psychology. Nor must we forget that the investigation of religious psychology was begun under the ægis of that scientific positivism which claims to be a systematic philosophy, an integral *Weltanschauung*. Renda, therefore, should not fail to recognize that the agnosticism favoured by Flournoy already represents a concession to antipositivistic criticism.

Let no one, therefore, be under any illusion : from the labour of sincere scientists we can obtain nothing but scientific convictions. Science aspires to tangible certainty, which is at once verifiable and universal. On that account it must necessarily be based on experience and, where necessary, upon logic as well, reducing faith (that is, personal assent not obviously suggested either by experience or by logic) to a minimum. Whoever seeks support for the thesis of idealism or of positivism, or awaits propulsion towards faith or estrangement from the religious spirit, is under a delusion. After psychology has done its work, he must solve his problems for himself ; whether by burying himself in the study of philosophy or naturalism, in idealism or neo-scholasticism ; or by abandoning himself to religious emotion.

None the less, it is to be clearly understood that the psychologist, having once taken up his stand on the basis of agnosticism, is in duty bound to consider religious phenomena not only or particularly from their external aspect, but he is also and especially bound to regard them as the processes of souls aflame with faith and imbued with a desire to possess absolute truth.

From the above considerations it will be clear that the psychologist who wishes to study religious phenomena in their descriptive, psycho-genetic, and physiological aspects, must adopt the methods and aim of Ribot and many American psychologists, such as Starbuck,[19] Royce, or William James.[20] But while avoiding any philosophical or theological bravado, he will also refrain from following recent tentatives such, for example, as those of the psychiatrist Binet-Sanglé [21] who has written on the *Folie de Jésus* (The Insanity of Jesus), or of that other celebrated psychologist, Stanley Hall, who in his book *Jesus the Christ in the Light of Psychology*, published in 1917, made a highly elaborate analysis of Christ.[22] Binet-Sanglé's book is the realization of an anti-Christian programme accomplished by means of a collection of historical documents and psychiatric illustrations, devoid of all critical spirit. The notable study of Stanley Hall is not only psychology; it is also history, theology, sociology and other things, with none of which we are concerned.

Here, however, we come upon psycho-analytic research as understood by Sigmund Freud,[23] which to-day extends into the sphere of religion and myth, on which, besides Freud, Rank and Reik have written. Psycho-analysis has been applied to the study of individual mystic and religious souls, and has also been used in the interpretation of ethnological and prehistoric material. Berguer has made a psycho-analysis of Jesus. Morel has psycho-analysed several of the Christian mystics; and this author has discovered that the fundamental psychic fact explaining these phenomena is *introversion*, in which the attention is diverted by an objective and by a repressed desire.[24] Others again of this school, as for example Rank and Reik,[25] have consulted historical documents or made ethnological investigations from which they claim to have discovered, through the psycho-analytic technique, the psychic basis of the origins of all religions.

The two modes of application of the methods of psycho-analysis are notably different. Psycho-analysis applied to the individual proceeds from his behaviour (his gestures, conversation, the accounts he gives of his dreams, etc.) to the psychological motivation of that behaviour—a motivation which, whenever possible, is verified by the conscious testimony of the individual himself, while being interrogated. The psycho-analyst,

after the verification, bases his findings on the psycho-
analytic interpretations which are fundamentally
doctrinaire ; that is to say, informed by a certain set
of general ideas, which, although originally founded on
empirical observations, have to-day almost assumed the
authority of principles. Everyone will agree that this
sort of application of the psycho-analytic technique,
though dangerous, is legitimate and full of promise.
On the other hand, the application of this method to
the investigation of the unconscious mind of a people,
through the psycho-analysis of its ritual, its ceremonials,
its behaviour, its customs, and by means of the study
of its cultural history, and so forth, is only a tacit
application of the results of individual analysis to race
psychology ; an interpretation of 'external' facts,
based upon the experience drawn from the psycho-
analysis of a few individuals, and availing itself of easy
generalizations. Even this may be good psychology ;
but there is no denying that these intuitions in respect
of origins appear much more laboured, and the applica-
tions of these doctrines much more daring.

The psycho-analytic method applied to race history,
in my opinion, can figure only as a 'control'—albeit
a valuable one—of other hypotheses, especially those of
sociology. Psycho-analysis may lead to new hypotheses ;
but these are only hypotheses, since they are not direct
statements of facts, but merely psychological interpretations of 'external' social phenomena, on the basis of
scanty observations, which in their turn have been
elaborated by means of an hypothesis ; and since these
interpretations are not susceptible of verification by the
testimony of the individual consciousness. Another
objection to such interpretations is that many philosophers,
anthropologists, and sociologists hold hypotheses widely

different from the Freudian explanations of the origin of religion and of myths.

The results obtained by psycho-analysis—which are certainly ingenious, although often one-sided—cannot, any more than these of sociology, provide workable interpretations of the various phenomena of religion, as, for example, conversion. This is because, in such cases, the consciousness of the subject lends value to the unconscious factor which is supposed to be the real fulcrum of the conversion. In reality, however, this factor need be no more than a common automatism, of a more or less remote instinctive origin ; it need only be a factor capable of acquiring a religious significance in the consciousness of the individual.

From all this two consequences ensue : the first is that contemporary religious psychology—in the sense adopted by Flournoy—has been assigned modest limits, which do not include history and sociology ; the second is that the scope and the field of action occupied by religious psychology are quite other than those of either ethnology or sociology.

It will readily be understood that this view cannot be pleasing to those sociologists who adhere more or less to the opinions of Durkheim.[26] It cannot be denied that the so-called sociological method, and the study of the folklore of various nations, may be capable of yielding an interpretation of ancient and modern religions, of the origins of myths and of cults, and of their ethical content.[27] It is, however, also true that all this throws no light on the religious soul of the individual, that is to say, the attitudes and emotions of believers.

There are those who believe that the effect of understanding the origin of a phenomenon is to make the soul ' indifferent ' to the phenomenon itself. Knowing is the

antithesis of feeling. To be sure, a child would not be
terrified by a phantasm or a tale if he could only understand how it happened to come into being. I myself have
experienced this state of mind, during mediumistic
séances, as soon as the weird movements and the strange
apparitions were recognized as the work of the medium.
But this is not altogether so in other spheres. An
anatomist, for instance, who knows the human skeleton
thoroughly, and the precise inter-relations of the muscles
of the thorax and the abdomen, is not thereby deprived
of one whit of æsthetic enjoyment of the Apollo Belvedere,
or the Hermes of Olympia. Does the reader imagine
that, because the surgeon is accustomed to the dissection
of every portion of the body, he is, on that account,
less emotionally susceptible to the beauty of the female
body than one who has no anatomical knowledge? I
have seen that the knowledge of the history of amulets
and the origins of superstitions does not destroy a
belief in the 'power' of the *jettatura* ('the evil eye').
No marvel, then, that the knowledge of the historical
origins of a ceremonial or a cult or an ascetic practice is
unable to annul the religious spirit. It may be that such
a knowledge refines and spiritualizes, while destroying
nothing.

There remains, however, a vast field for psychological
research, after history and sociology have been excluded.
Thus, by the study of the individual mind, the psychologist can — if ever — understand race-history. Every
one of us, in his own person, can verify the worth of
many hypotheses concerning religion and the Divine.
Fundamentally it is the individual who has created the
ethnological and sociological theories of the various
religions. Indeed an empirical realist could declare

that objective science, after all, is only the objectivation of the subjective.

The field of action of religious psychology must be internal experience considered in relation to the behaviour (to which it is correlative) of the individual or of the religious group.[28] The various methods and processes of religious psychology are those—and none other than those—of contemporary psychology, whether analytic, synthetic, or differential, and especially those of voluntary introspection and induced introspection, questioning and external observation.

Various psychologists have already attempted to establish a psychological method and a technique applicable to the investigation of religious phenomena. We find Wundt in the forefront, with his *Völkerpsychologie* ; then follow Stanley Hall and Starbuck, with their methods of the questionnaire and of statistics ; and lastly and above all, there is James, with empirical research directly applied to the religious consciousness. But the scope of this work precludes us from examining the merits and faults of the various individual methods adopted by the psychologists of religion, which, moreover, the recent excellent critique by Georg Wobbermin [29] makes superfluous.

A modest task is that here proposed ; and to those who, because of its agnosticism and of its limitations, would accuse contemporary religious psychology of sterility, we would reply that this is far from being the opinion of modern theologians, whether Protestants or Catholics. At any rate, it is not the view of those who, like Truc, Huby,[30] Monsignore Sturzo,[31] and other critics of the doctrine of *l'educateur invisible* of Father Mainage, show a tendency to delimit with an even greater rigour the ambit of ' grace ', or to study ' grace ' psychologically. For

them certain phenomena, which were once regarded as
transcendental, are active and personal, and as such
psychological *par excellence*,[32] even if the believer thinks
himself guided by Divine Providence or ' grace '. All
this, indeed, implies that it is not useless to try to
establish, by all the resources of modern psychology,
the working, in conversion and in other religious
phenomena, of those processes which we understand
by the conception and the term ' personal will '. The
psychologist, confronted by the simple attitude of
those who attribute all our mutations to ' grace ', must
not forget the words in St. Matthew, xi, 12 : "Until
now the kingdom of heaven suffereth violence, and the
violent take it by force."

Indeed, I am persuaded after voluminous reading
on the subject of conversion, that even the religious
leaders are beginning to regard and study conversion
in a way very different from that of former times. I
have especially remarked that the conversions described
in the old books, for example, were, almost without
exception, referred to some external cause. They were
attributed to marvels of all sorts, to exhortations and
prophecies on the part of missionaries or priests
(*piscatores hominum*), to apparitions, arguments, books,
dreams, to tempests, chance encounters, and diverse
accidents ; and this as much in collective as in individual
conversions.[33]   To-day, unless I deceive myself, even the
apologists show a much finer intuition in explaining
and commenting on conversions occurring in our own
times. This is a sign that psychological culture, even
in them, has made no little progress.[34]

The theme of conversion, after that of ecstasy, is
probably the best known in the psychology of mysticism

and religion. I do not refer to the phenomena of mass-conversion, which have occurred in all ages, and of which there are still manifestations at the present time; for these are social phenomena of complex origin. Since my especial task is to elucidate the process of conversion, I am occupied only with the conversion of individuals free from external influences of too general and too obvious a nature.

It formerly seemed that after Pascal, Bossuet, and Fénélon, little could be added to the subject of conversion. But romanticism first and then the psychological sciences have—so to speak—revived the fashion for analysis of the converted and of those ' called '. So much so, that to-day we have a psychology of vocation [35] and a vast literature on the subject of conversion. After Newman's *Apologia*, there appeared from opposite camps the *Bonne Souffrance* of François Coppée, and William James's *Varieties of Religious Experience*. Then followed the investigations of the American psychologists, Leuba's studies,[36] and the psychological analysis of the testimony, written or oral, of the converts themselves. And lastly we have psycho-analysis according to the technical methods and doctrines of Freud.

That I take part in this discussion is due chiefly to the fact that I have before me the unpublished evidence of several converts. Among these, in particular, is that of a young Anglican (Case No. 1), of two atheists or rationalists (Cases 2 and 3), and of a Jewish lady (Case 4), who have all embraced Catholicism with sincerity and constancy.

In connection with conversion there arise a number of questions of general analytic psychology, and especially of individual psychology.

A German convert to Catholicism, Kurt Rothe,[37] in an important lecture delivered in 1921, attempted to reduce the processes of conversion, so widely divergent in individual instances, to a certain normal standardization of types (or *Typisierung*, to use the convenient German term). I myself had made an attempt at such a classification, before Rothe, but after a different method and with different results. However that may be, it is undeniable that the various modes of religious conversion may differ vastly in different groups of individuals.[38] Huysmans himself, in his *Pages Catholiques*, has enumerated three distinct types.

In this book I propose to take soundings here and there in the vast sea of this subject, in order to show, if possible, the intimate process of what we may term *the typical experience of conversion.*

CHAPTER II

CONVERSION AND ITS CAUSES

BEFORE proceeding further it is essential to come to
some agreement as to the meaning of the term
conversion. It is frequently employed not only in theology,
but in logic ('the conversion of propositions'), in
arithmetic, and in finance. A few remarks are therefore
necessary, in order to avoid the risk of introducing
an equivocal term into modern psychology.

In connection with the psychology of memory,
Professor J. M. Baldwin has made considerable use of
the term 'conversion'.[1] This distinguished psychologist
has, as is well known, made a study, in memory, of the
genetic development of knowledge. Memory has the
characteristic of representing something : it is a *mode
of representation*. But it has a second characteristic ;
namely, that it remains subject to the control of a more
or less remote sensory context, rather than to the
immediate control of the actual sensory context. From
this point of view, therefore, memory is a *mode of
conversion*. The object of memory becomes 'converted'
over again into an object of the senses. It is a 'conversion of return'. In its fullest sense, the index
of the control of memory is the 'convertibility' of a
context. The objects of memory always remain representational ; they are always 'convertible', and always
subject to direct control. The recollection of any event
always implies the same context as that of the original

event, and always implies the ' conversion ' of the original
experience into a renewed experience. In this theory,
the word ' conversion ' has the precise meaning of
' renewal ', by means of a return to the original source.

Since the researches of Freud, however, the word
' conversion ' may be found in pathological psychology,
where it has naturally acquired an entirely different
significance. ' Conversion hysteria ' (*Konversionshysterie*) [2]
means the transformation of an unconscious psychic
·content into a phenomenon of the somatic sphere,
such as a tic, convulsions, or other visible disturbances.
In this sense, the term ' conversion ' implies a mutation
from psychic to somatic phenomena which are equivalent
or, better, correlative.

It might be imagined that the meaning of conversion
in religious psychology would be identical with that in
theology. This is not altogether so, because in theology
conversion comprises a variety of shades of meaning
under a single term. Thus conversion in the Acts of the
Apostles comprises not only the sense of repentance,
but also of faith in Jesus Christ ; in theology conversion
is defined in terms of the two elements of which it consists,
' grace ' and aspiration. Moreover, from the fourth
century till the seventh, what was called conversion
was, in fact, the ' renunciation of the life of this world ',
in order to devote oneself to the sacred orders, or the
monastic regime. Hence the term *conversi* or *frati
conversi* in distinction to the *oblati*.

In current usage, among Catholic writers on matters
ecclesiastical, conversion ordinarily means a passage
from unbelief (or from a non-Catholic religion) to Roman
Catholicism. The same term, however, has come to be
adopted also in the case of a reversion or ' return '
to that religion after a longer or shorter period of

wandering from its precepts. It is also employed to denote cases of 'acknowledgment' or 'recognition' (of Catholicism) after many years of religious indifference. The term conversion (in German: *Bekehrung*) has— it must be clearly understood—also been adopted into the terminology of other religions outside the pale of Catholicism. But in the non-Catholic, English-speaking countries conversion acquires a special meaning, of which we shall take account later on.

In religious psychology, conversion implies 'mutation', not of cult, but rather of conscience, regarding the sentiment and practice of a religion.

There are frequently philosophico-moral conversions as well as those of religion and cult. These, however, must be kept distinct, although they contain certain elements in common with the former group. For instance, the philosophical and moral conversions effected by Seneca—a true spiritual director—are not in all respects comparable to religious conversions, although that philosopher, when Lucilius, who had been an Epicurean, became a temperate Stoic, recommended to him even poverty, as Epictetus had previously done in his *Encheiridion*.[3] In the period of revulsion against the corruption of manners and of exhaustion after the breakdown of the Roman power, nobler souls turned towards philosophy in the same spirit as that which animated Livia, the wife of Augustus, after the loss of Drusus.

But a little reflection shows that these spiritual attitudes were merely aspirations towards the attainment of an immediate peace, or towards the achievement of a death without fear. Religion, on the contrary, whether it be specific or generic ('religiousness') necessarily implies 'values', which are more universal, transcendent, and

immortal. Philosophical and moral conversions, therefore, cannot legitimately be included within the scope
of the present work, even when they contain both the
theory and the practice of a higher ideal.

The religious Neo-Platonism of Julian the Apostate
was a philosophic initiation ; it was no actual conversion,
although the mystic soul of the pupil of Iamblichus and
of Maximus of Ephesus burned with a lively faith in its
own mission.

A certain stir was made in Paris some thirty years ago
by the conversion to theosophical mysticism of a
materialistic and evolutionist doctor, known under
the pseudonym of ' Dr. Papus '. Reflection made him
recognize that an important factor was being neglected
in the evolutionary theory. Evolution he admitted ;
but he held that it was necessary for the physico-chemical
forces and those of the sun to reinforce evolution ; that
is, the superior forces in evolution sacrifice themselves
for the evolution of the inferior forces. Thus, while the
theory of evolution brought to light the law of the
struggle for existence, was there not another law, co-
existing and forgotten, the law of sacrifice ? It chanced
one day that the doctor discovered that these deductions
were old and that they could all be found in ancient
occultism and in alchemy ; and, by reading, he convinced
himself of the analogical method which allowed of the
unification of all the sciences into a common synthesis.
Thus ' Dr. Papus ' became a convert to occultism.[4]
Now such a mutation truly possesses the character of
a religious conversion, but we can see, none the less,
how difficult it would be actually to identify it with
conversion. On this account, it cannot be included
as one of the typical cases of religious conversion best
suited to psychological analysis.

Starbuck distinguishes *counter-conversions* from true conversions. The notable case of the French philosopher Jouffroy, described at length by James, is typical.[5] But this author also refers to other cases, all of the 'lightning' or fulminant type. Counter-conversion indicates the passage from some religious creed to free-thought. Literature gives us a well-known example of this type in Emile Zola's Pierre Froment.

The philosopher Roberto Ardigò was a convert from Catholicism to positivism, or better, a counter-convert— so much so that Gaetano Negri has compared his mutation to that of St. Paul. It was said that his mutation was unforeseen, and occurred while the philosopher was observing a rose. It seems, however, that the instanta- neousness claimed by Gaetano Negri and the rest at the time of the occurrence should be extended to a period of forty days to accord with the facts, unless we are ready to accept the unworthy suggestion that Canon Ardigò changed his religion because his superiors had wounded his pride. The psychologist would have to study the documents of the case in order to define the exact conversional processes of the philosopher. But however we may regard it, we must exclude Ardigò's case from the present inquiry because it is a case of a purely intellectual mutation—as everyone agrees—and Ardigò's life, that is to say, his sentiments and morals, remained unchanged. For this reason it must be excluded also from the classification of counter-conversion. It is much more probable that in Ardigò there occurred, as a result of his studies of positivism, a mutation of his philosophical convictions (one recalls his dissertation on Pomponazzi, for which he was suspended *a divinis*), a mutation which he manifested regardless of con- sequences, as his rectitude counselled.

Neither are the changes in conduct of many American alcoholics, included in Starbuck's inquiry, to be considered as true conversions; nor are those of the Welsh drunkards who were 'converted' during the famous Revivals,[6] though it is impossible to deny that such changes of conduct have great ethical value. Often these consist merely in moral mutations or at the very most—at least in certain instances—in 'returns', or in 'recognitions' which are more or less permanent.

Some publicity has recently been given to the conversion of the writer Giosuè Borsi; but this case seems to have been merely one of 'recognition'.[7]

It is very difficult to distinguish in particular cases true and genuine conversion—which is an overturning of values—from 'recognition' and 'return'. Thus the commoner cases consist mainly in a 'conscious return' to the faith and habits of childhood, in defence of threatened personal values; or in unconscious 'transferences' of the imaginative and affective energy liberated from representational systems, which have become weakened because unserviceable, on to older objects of consciousness.

The conversation of François Coppée was evidently a case of such a return to faith. During the crises of his adolescence he had discarded devotional exercises, but had never actually rejected his beliefs. "*Oui*," he writes in *La Bonne Souffrance*, "*plus j'y songe, plus je crois qu'un peu de foi chrétienne sommeilla toujours au fond de mon cœur.*"

The conversion of Primot,[8] as described by himself, was, perhaps, another such return. He had been religious during the period of his first youth and then became a positivist, remaining so up to his forty-fifth year. At this age he gave himself up to the study of the great problems of philosophy, and after passing through a phase of spiritualism, made his return to religious belief at the age of sixty.

A distinction must be made between conversion and 'development' in the psychical, and more especially in the moral, sense. Some authorities have spoken of what they call 'conversion by development', by which they mean that the fact of conversion is the final phase of the 'typical' evolution of the mind or the soul. It seems to me difficult to consider cases of this sort as actual conversions. Let us take Goethe's Marguerite as an example. When she had passed through her trials, after her brother's curses, after her sufferings in prison, she redeemed herself from the senses and resisted first Faust who wanted to save her, and finally Mephistopheles. This does not seem to me to be a conversion. Suffering having removed the obstacles, this woman's soul, purified of passion, once more resumed the ways into which it was initiated in early childhood. This appears, therefore, a true 'development', and not an overturning of values nor a true *Metanoia*.

Even less do the so-called 'crises of conscience' deserve to be classified as conversions, crises such as occur in the lives of politicians who change sides from conservatism to socialism, or *vice versa*.

There are, too, many illusory conversions and many abortive conversions which have failed to mature. Once the poet Verlaine believed he was converted, and Pierre Loti and Maurice Barrès seem to have started out in this direction.[9]

Our present theme is, however, limited to the consideration of such conversions as are genuine, complete, and lasting. We wish to regard the phenomena of conversion from the strictly religious angle. We do not share the opinion of some who would restrict conversion to Catholicism, since true and fully-established moral conversions—or mutations of life under the impulse of an ultra-terrestrial ideal—are to be found, not only in paganism, but in all times and among all peoples, no matter what their religion. But, in order to sound the fullest depths of our subject, it is essential to offer facts in evidence, and the author believes that the Catholic religion offers the richest yield of facts. However that may be, I intend to refer, almost exclusively, to phenomena connected with the Catholic religion.

But while thus restricting ourselves, we must insist that this study makes no claim to exhaust the subject. Here we attempt merely to examine the *most typical experiences* of those converted to Catholicism. We are compelled to leave aside such conversions as deserve to be called *atypical* in relation to our own selected type, and all the lengthy series of individual variations from either of these groups.

At the very outset we must examine the first phase of the process which takes place in cases of conversion. We must consider the *ætiology of conversion*.

The positivists insist upon stressing the *physiological causes* of conversion. Among these they mention nervous or mental disorders ; exhausting diseases, such as tuberculosis ; special conditions, such as puberty and senility, with the inevitable cerebral disabilities peculiar to the latter period. Here and there may be found such cases of a purely physiological ætiology of conversion. But, up to the present, one must say that the physiological factors that are met with in the antecedent circumstances of any given series of converts, always appear to have required a psychic factor for their effective development. For example, we have cerebral arterio-sclerosis accompanied by mental deficiency ; toxæmias accompanied by melancholia or mania ; organic exhaustion accompanied by an increase of suggestibility, and so forth.

The crux of the controversy, however, does not lie here, nor in the fact of the existence of some disorder in the nervous system of the convert, but rather in the relations existing between conversion and the disease. Without stopping here to go into all the details of the argument, it suffices to say that there is no necessary or essential connection.

Old age as a factor of conversion has been admitted by the uninformed ; but the so-called conversions among the senile—and to an even greater degree, among the dying—are only very rarely typical conversions, according to the standards which we have laid down. They are more correctly to be classified as ' regressions ' or ' returns ' to faith.

Among the mentally diseased and the neurasthenics conversional processes may indeed occur, but, as we have already stated, these processes have characteristics which differ from those of the normal individual. Indeed, when we examine cases of true conversion, we find that the disorder is not the necessary antecedent, in other words it is not what is known as the cause.

Puberty as a cause of conversion has been given considerable prominence by the American school of psychologists, particularly by Starbuck and Stanley Hall, who have published statistics and discussed the problem.

According to the American psychologists, conversion is a natural phenomenon of adolescence. They regard it as a purely normal and almost universal accompaniment of the epoch in life when the personality becomes hetero-centric. In support of this, Starbuck, Daniells, and other observers declare that eighty per cent of all conversions occur during adolescence. The age-period of highest frequency, according to some of these observers (D. L. Moody and M. S. Kees), is between the tenth and the twentieth years. By other statisticians it is placed after the fifteenth year. In a statistical table of the results of an inquiry by Stanley Hall,[10] the highest frequency of conversion for both sexes is given as occurring between the eleventh and the twenty-third years. Other authorities give the mean age of conversion among women as fourteen years and eight months, and among men as sixteen years and four months. George A. Coe is of opinion that at the age of thirteen occur the first stirrings towards conversion ; at seventeen a second impulse occurs ; and the maximum is reached at the age of twenty. Before the age of twelve, according to Lancaster, religion is a mere form.

According to Starbuck, who is probably the most authoritative investigator in this field, conversion occurs almost exclusively between the ages of ten and twenty-five ; whence it would follow that it is a phenomenon characteristic of the age of development of the organism and the mind. If conversion has not taken place before the twentieth year, there is little probability that it will come later.

In women the curve of frequency begins to ascend at the age of ten and continues to rise till thirteen. It falls after this age till fifteen, and culminates at the age of sixteen. (This was the age at which forty of the three hundred selected cases were converted.) It sinks again at seventeen, but has a fresh rise at eighteen, after which it falls gradually to the age of twenty. The maxima of frequency, therefore, are observable at the ages of thirteen, sixteen, and eighteen years. In male subjects the curve starts as early as nine. It rises at twelve and falls at thirteen. It again mounts suddenly at sixteen, the age at which it culminates ; but it still remains high till, at nineteen, it drops. The maxima of male conversions are seen at the ages of twelve, sixteen, and nineteen years of age.

Starbuck concludes from these data that there must be a physiological cause for the process of conversion, since it coincides with the period of most rapid bodily development. However, as this author points out, though there are numerous conversions during the period of puberty, the most conspicuous phenomena of puberty itself do not coincide with the most frequent conversions.

Stanley Hall endeavours to discover the homology of religious conversion in nature and finds its equivalent in the metamorphoses of insects and in other zoological mutations.[11] Everyone can recognize that such remotely distant analogies are so strained as to be scarcely worth mentioning. In my opinion, conversion (in the American sense) in its biological aspect can only be interpreted as a phenomenon of ' adaptation for defence ', and (in the sense here adopted) it is a phenomenon of the renewal of life and of ' regeneration '.

In regard to the physiological aspect of adolescent mutations, we may speak more precisely. The glands of internal secretion are especially active throughout the whole of adolescence, which is the period attended by the most active organic transformations.[12] It will be easily recognized that the establishment of this fact is not without significance for all who—like ourselves— find at the root of the processes of conversion a mutation of sexual economy.

Nevertheless, although these facts and the American statistics are of great interest for those who would study religious phenomena from the biological aspect, the data should be accepted with due reserve.

What are we to assume that Starbuck and the American school in general mean by the term 'conversion'? Apparently nothing beyond the moral and religious crisis of adolescence.   It should be remembered that these conversions of the epoch of puberty which Starbuck has studied, refer to youths educated in an evangelical community. Becoming 'converted' for these youths means to be freed from their doubts and their scruples, and from painful moral conflicts in general.   Such 'conversions' are liberations influenced by that increase of faith in themselves which results from the psychic development so exuberantly manifested on the threshold of youth. One must further add that the American psychologists treat conversion exclusively from the ethical standpoint, which makes it simpler than ever to take into account the modifications of the moral sentiments and of the individual conduct of the subject which occur under the influence of a religious education once the subject has reached the age of puberty, with all its attendant intellectual and sexual crises. Moreover, the contrary phenomena are also frequent— perhaps even more frequent—at this period. It is an undoubted fact that during puberty many youths undergo a crisis of religious indecision or of actual unbelief (between fifteen and sixteen years of age according to Stanley Hall) and even a crisis of criminality.

Cesare Lombroso and A. Marro noted these alterations in emotion and conduct during the period of puberty, and the observations and statistics which they published in this connection are of the highest interest.[13] The literature of the past few years has confirmed the great frequency of moral delinquency among minors; and from the most recent Italian statistics it is evident that juvenile delinquents have been steadily on the increase since 1891, and that this increase has continued; after the outbreak of the War it reached alarming proportions, as shown by the total figures relating to convictions under eighteen as well as by percentages; and there are indications that since the War there has been no diminution in this direction.

It must be added that counter-conversions during the period of puberty and adolescence are of frequent occurrence, especially among students, and are largely determined by the preponderance of the sexual instinct. The words of St. Augustine are still applicable to such cases. In fact we must conclude that the period between the ages of fifteen and twenty-five is the time when the greatest changes occur in human personality, and therefore that this is the epoch most propitious for the occurrence of decisive events in the history of individuals. We also see confirmation of this from the American statistics of immigration; from figures dealing with the selection of trades and professions; from the statistics of marriages and of the age-incidence of tuberculosis.

These considerations, in my opinion, clarify the ætiological significance of the period of adolescence as a factor in religious conversion. We are here dealing only with an extrinsic or indirect cause, neither essential nor sufficient; in other words, with a provocative stimulus to an intellectual and ethical transformation which becomes effective only in certain individuals, and only under determined psychic and environmental conditions.

It need hardly be added that conversion has not quite the same significance for the writer as for the American psychologists. For them conversion is merely a feature of the curve of the normal moral development in those who from youth receive in the American colleges an education influenced by the spirit of religion. For us, on the other hand, conversion is an exceptional process experienced in adolescence or maturity, and representing an intellectual and moral regeneration of the person in whom it occurs. And further, conversion is a process which may be observed in anyone whatsoever ; in those who have undergone the so-called ethico-religious conversion of adolescence, as well as in those who have been unbelieving or immoral from childhood, or in those who have remained throughout indifferent to religion. This means that conversion—in our sense—has an ætiology far too complex to allow us to ascribe it to disease, age, endocrine variations, or the like.

After this consideration of the general *physiological* causes of conversion, we now examine its *psychic* causes.

The external psychic causes are very frequently indicated by authors who treat of religious conversion, but it must be remembered that these could not have been effective without the antecedent, simultaneous, or subsequent occurrence of internal psychic causes. As in every psychic process, the initial stimulus is to be sought outside consciousness ; but without the interior elaboration of the stimulus—an elaboration which, as we shall see later, is not entirely unconscious—the process would never develop.

Many and various are the stimuli which may provoke the process of conversion. There is suggestion, in the form of sermons, missions, and reading ; example, such as that found in the testimony of the confessors and martyrs ; marvellous happenings, such as prophecies and miracles ; occult and mediumistic practices ; politico-social propaganda ; æsthetic stimulation ; the ardours of nationalism ; misfortunes and illnesses ; the great cosmic or social calamities, from earthquakes to wars and revolutions—all of which become effective by means of elaboration in the individual consciousness.[14]

Collective conversions, resulting from a different series of factors and often difficult of analysis, are phenomena of great importance from the historical and sociological aspect. There are, for instance, the mass-conversions to Christianity brought about by missionaries among uncivilized communities, especially in Africa ; those, too, evoked by the ethico-mystical movement of the so-called Revivals ; those which frequently occur in non-Catholic countries to Roman Catholicism ; and the numerous and frequently collective conversions seen in Russia, in Germany, and elsewhere after the War and during the revolutions, and so forth.[15]

To us, however, even more interesting than these collective conversions are the conversions of individuals, since they lend themselves so much more fully to analysis.

The conversion of the two ' noble students ' of the Marches of Ancona, performed by St. Francis of Assisi in the course of his preachings at Bologna,[16] which is mentioned in the *Fioretti*, is an example of conversion by an external cause. Similarly, the mutation of the convert who afterwards became the Friar Bernard of Scesi, the first companion of St. Francis, was due to the impression made by St. Francis during one night when he lodged in his house.

Again, the conversion of the fourteenth-century mystic, the Blessed Giovanni Colombini, was brought about through the reading of the biography of St. Mary of Egypt who, according to the legend, had been a death-snare stretched for the souls of all men, but afterwards became " the woman submerged in grace and in love ".[17]

In San Marco in Florence, numerous mass-conversions resulted from the preaching of Savonarola, but even more interesting, for those who are studying the ætiology of religious mutations, are the individual conversions he produced. There was that of ' Bettuccio ', the son of a goldsmith, who was a miniature painter, a singer, and a poet. This convert had been an evil-liver, an unbeliever, and a partisan of the Arrabbiati against the Piagnoni, as Villari relates.[18] This was a characteristic example of conversion by suggestion. At the same time it shows how the phenomenon can disappear and recur ; and how too this conversion had, in common with so many psycho-physiological phenomena, a phase of secondary oscillations.

Bonajuti has described from an historical point of view the conversion of St. Augustine. The external ætiological elements of this conversion were the perusal of the ' Hortensius ', the words of St. Ambrose, and the retreat into the quiet solitude of Cassiciaco.[19]

One finds cases of conversions following a dream. But more frequently a ' call ' is heard during dreams, like that of the Emperor John of Constantinople who became a Frater Minor, under the influence of three dreams on three consecutive nights.[20] The ' call ' pre-supposes an interior preparation much more remarkable, and indeed much more conscious, than the conversion itself. In every instance, these dreams in their turn require a causal factor which is to be sought among the psychic stimuli of the subconscious, or in repressed desires.

Among the causes of religious conversions 'auto-imitation' deserves a place. This practice, indeed, was recommended to unbelievers by Pascal, in that celebrated passage of his *Pensées* well known in literature under the name of *pari de Pascal*.[21] By acquiring the habit of attending divine service, without any explicit purpose, faith is gradually acquired.

The philosopher Lutoslawski, of whom we shall have occasion to speak further later on, expounded to the Geneva Congress in 1909 his own special technique in the procedure necessary for the conversion of intellectuals. His method was not original; it was, indeed, a reproduction of the famous method of Pascal. We are not aware of any conversions which have been accomplished by this means. But even supposing that conversions have been thus effected, who can fail to perceive that this procedure of Pascal's presupposes the existence of faith, and that his method only serves to put the reason to sleep, leaving faith an unopposed efficacy? We are dealing, then, not with the cause of conversion, but with conversion itself.

In one of my own cases, conversion began by attending Catholic churches. But my convert, who had been an Anglican, observed: "Even before conversion I experienced great pleasure in finding myself in a church of the Catholic religion." Not habit, therefore, but the pleasure of forming the habit, began the conversional process. It can be easily understood that participation in the sacraments, and the performance of the simple ceremonies which belong to the cult, assist in producing a complete conversion, and once the conversion is effected, strengthen it powerfully, as in the case of my Anglican, and many other converts. Such cases we must regroup under the so-called ' cyclic law ', since a circle is evidently formed between action and thought so that both are at once mutually cause and effect.

Catholic ceremonial attracts not a few souls from Lutheranism to the worship of traditional Christianity. The Catholic liturgy, for example, played a considerable part in the conversion of the Dutchman Pieter van der Meer de Walcheren [22] as well as in that of Huysmans. My own first convert and my third both felt the mystic and æsthetic fascination of the vast and solitary nave and of the chanting of the liturgy.

I have learnt through the oral communications of competent witnesses that in England a certain proportion of conversions to Catholicism have been due to the unity of doctrine and of moral conduct of those who profess it. I have become convinced that during the War a large number of English soldiers were converted through being impressed by the uniformity of the faith and the moral precepts of the Catholic military chaplains attached to the various armies. It would also seem that in England the example of Cardinal Newman has always been a powerful stimulus towards conversion.

I found, in two cases, a return to Catholicism of persons who only believed in spiritism. One of those himself told me : " Spiritism was what persuaded me that Christ is God and that the Church is immortal." The conversion of the young woman described in *Les voies de Dieu* by Madame Mink-Jullien had its point of departure in the practices of occultism,[23] and that of Primot in spiritism, or, to use his own expression, experimental psychology.

It is commonly known that the teachings of

humanitarianism have sufficed for the conversion of
certain socialists of high principles to Catholicism.
An instance in point is the case of Don Camelli of Cremona,
who gives his own testimony of conversion in his book,
Dal Socialismo al Sacerdozio.[24]   In connection with
nationalism, also, a number of French converts have
declared that their return to Catholicism was the outcome
of the patriotic exaltation of the War.

Physical and moral suffering is, however, the miracle-
working external condition of religious conversion.

St. Francis of Assisi, as we shall see later, had during
the convalescence of a serious illness his first intimations
of his change towards God.   He felt much disquietude
and desired to leave at once for Apulia and enrol himself
as a soldier under the command of Walter III, Count
of Brienne and Champagne.   But when he reached
Spoleto he had a relapse, and it was in that illness that
he became definitely converted, his heart turning
permanently towards God and Poverty.

It was the realization that Louis XIV was gradually
abandoning her that first prepared the way of Madame
de la Vallière's soul towards God.   But it was a serious
illness that ultimately influenced this great courtesan
to seek the peace of the cloister.   While in a church at
Ems, in 1847, the final transformation of the celebrated
Jewish convert, Hermann Cohen, took place.   But he
had long been so markedly depressed, that they called
him the 'melancholy Puzzi'.   The conversion of the
famous Englishman, who afterwards became Cardinal
Newman, was preceded by years of interior conflict and
psychic depression, to such a degree that, according to
Brémond, his anxiety and disquietude counted for
important determining factors of his conversion.   The
compelling force of suffering is paramount in the con-

version of François Coppée. A disease necessitating frequent operations is acknowledged by the poet himself as the cause of his return to the faith and the resumption of his religious duties. This he confesses on several occasions, and especially in *La Meilleure Année (La Bonne Souffrance)*. If Elizabeth Leseur,[25] before her great physical sufferings, was influenced by education and by witnessing the religious rites of a conversion in 1903, certainly Felix Leseur, though to some degree influenced by his wife's example, was much more profoundly influenced by the immense sorrow of losing her. Even in so-called 'intellectual' conversions we see the same note of sadness during the early phases. This is evident in connection with the conversions of Puel de Lobel, Pierre de Lescure, and in the case of the highly intellectual André de Bavier, of whom Mainage writes : " Even he needed to feel the heavy hand of suffering weighing upon him." Robert Hugh Benson found in the death of his father the decisive impulse which made him enter the Church of Rome.

Certainly the study of literature and the facts of my own experience furnish convincing evidence that before an adult turns towards religious faith he must have undergone the experience of suffering. (I do not here include the adolescent, because I do not possess the necessary documentary support.) Whether it be the experience of illness, mutilation, imprisonment, or hunger, or some domestic misfortune, or moral perturbation, it is indisputable that every true conversion has suffering for its antecedent. It may even be that suffering is the one indispensable factor, although suffering alone is insufficient. For the rest, the same phenomenon is apparent in mass-conversions. The War with its aftermath of ruin and desolation, economic and moral depression, the overturning of the standards of value of a people—these are among the powerful influences which result in numerous returns to the faith.

How often it happens that the most lofty minds, saddened by the contemplation of the sorrows of others, and reflecting them in the mirror of their sensitive souls, gladly abandon themselves to religious belief. This is borne out by the following personal testimony of Giovanni Papini: "At last I was convinced that all the attempts which men made to institute an ephemeral felicity on earth were pitiable failures and were only successful in sowing blood and tears. It then appeared to me that the one channel of escape from all our misery is offered by the unheeded words of Christ. So I drew near to the Gospels with my heart full of hope and love." [26]

When we allude to sorrowful experiences we reach the most profound of all the *internal* causes of conversion. Indeed, all who show signs of radical mutations of personality will have already experienced a more or less conscious internal crisis.

Running through the literature, one often finds that before the conversion the subject was in some exceptional organic condition. This may have been determined either by external events or by some state of the body itself. But in certain cases these organic predisposing conditions are absent. Instead, conversion is suddenly ushered in by a complete alteration of character, or else by the appearance of some urgent moral need, in short, with new psychic dispositions of the subject. These phenomena are described in the autobiographies—when they have been consciously felt—by a variety of terms. We read, for instance, of the need of a doctrinal system ; or of a sure mental and moral direction ; or

of the want of superior aid. We hear of the delusions
of this world; of a craving for an outlet for activity;
of disgust at physical pleasures; sometimes of the need
for love.   More generally there exists a state of
anxiety of the intelligence and of the soul. Conversion
accordingly appears to the 'predestined'—in its
intellectual aspect—as an affirmation after a series of
negations; and—from the affective aspect—as the
conquest of equilibrium, of peace and joy. The convert
finally 'knows', and is at last serene.

Cardinal Newman was drawn towards Catholicism
by an imperative need for mental order; for a system of
dogma. The Rev. Frederick Joseph Kinsman, former
Bishop of the Episcopal Church of Delaware,[27] has stated
in his recent book that his 'genuine conversion' came
about very gradually. As he became slowly convinced
that the Catholic Church was the best of all institutions,
he acknowledged the doctrine of the supremacy of the
Church herself as integral and essential.

Men of letters, such as Paul Bourget, Jules Bois, and
probably Huysmans and others, deliberately returned
again to religion through a crisis of the will; through
the conscious need of mental direction. In my third
case the convert, a man of science, unable to discover
in science a foundation on which to base a strong
conviction, was happy to find such a foundation in
revealed truth, and in the authority of the Church.

It appears that St. Augustine himself experienced
this overpowering need when he wrote the words: " I
would not lend faith even to the gospel, if thou, O
Catholic Church, didst not command it of me." [28]

Moreover, these crises of moral need are frequently
to be observed among habitual criminals. Manzoni's
' Innominato ' is such a type in art.[29] The alcoholics

of America, of whom Starbuck speaks, and the Welsh of the Revivals, are common examples in everyday life. Outside the bounds of the Catholic Church, we have the famous case of the alcoholic S. H Hadley, described by William James.

An intellectual moment is certainly a stage in the conversional process; and it can be clearly discerned as a particular state of logical conviction, among the causes determining a conversion. It is incontestable, however, that, consciously or otherwise, the conversion is always initiated in an affective moment. How else can we explain the cases of certain extraordinary conversions to Catholicism, which the subjects themselves have attributed to Darwinism, like that of Jœrgensen; to the reading of Schopenhauer, like that of Hermann Ronge (the imaginary hero of Jœrgensen) [30]; or to the reading of *Port Royal* by Sainte Beuve?

When describing their conversions, converts do not always exactly reproduce their actual experiences. If, however, their writings are carefully read—or better still, if they themselves can be personally interrogated— the reality becomes apparent. Even among converts from Protestantism, Newman, Robert Hugh Benson, André de Bavier, and Kinsman, all of whom would appear to be classic examples of conversion for intellectual reasons—we discover expressions of a passionate devotion to the Roman Church, which they insistently call ' Mother ' or ' Queen ', who " knows how to single out and draw aside the least among her sons, and to feel their sorrows ".[31]

For the rest, such converts themselves recognize an emotional tumult as an immediate antecedent of their mutations. This perhaps may be the appropriate place in which to mention the confession of profound sadness

E

of the philosopher Jouffroy at the moment of his counter-conversion.   We have, too, the very important testimony of Lutoslawski of Cracow, another converted philosopher, who thus expressed himself at the Congress of Psychology at Geneva : [32] " This faith has become the whole centre of the work of adapting my philosophical convictions to the dogma of the Church Universal . . . But my conversion was not above all a change of conviction.   It was essentially a change of attitude, of the direction of my will ; a resolution to live within the Church and to unite myself with Christ manifest in the Sacrament.   The system of my metaphysical convictions was in no way shattered by my conversion."

The so-called psychic states preceding conversion seem all to have this in common, that they dissolve the economy of the individual, and excite the soul, but cannot satisfy it or allay its disturbance.   They are psychic states which propound questions, but do not answer them ; they initiate, but do not complete.   They provoke a suspension of the soul in which they are being experienced· This is the reason why all converts express themselves as happy after the crisis.   *Facta est (in eis) tranquillitas magna*.   We seem to hear the words of Dante :—

> *Quinci si va chi vuol andar per pace.*
> (*Purg.* XXIV, 141.) *

It is a state of the soul which is never absent—as has already been remarked—even in converts who experience as the initial stage of their psychic change a new conviction, that is, an intellectual element.   Bishop Kinsman confesses in his autobiography that the only sentiment he can recall having after his conversion is one of contentment.   Having found " the true ark of

* " Hence goeth he who desires to go for peace."

salvation ", every personal desire was satisfied. "The kingdom of heaven," he says, " is a pearl of great price." Monsignor Benson, too, confesses that he felt a kind of contented tranquillity that increased within his heart, almost instant by instant.

It is curious how much more rarely than one would expect the internal cause of the conversion is ascribed to the fear of damnation. This fear, however, is clearly implicit, inasmuch as salvation is regarded as of supreme worth by the convert, and the kingdom of heaven is the " pearl of great price " ; yet the fact remains, the fear of damnation does not find explicit expression—which implies that it is not in consciousness—among the confessions of true converts.

It is worth noting, on the other hand, that the fear of death and the dread of the Beyond is the foremost cause of the conversion of the old and the sick. But these ' conversions ' are more accurately classified as returns in old age from indifference to the sacraments.

In the Chapter which follows, I shall further develop what—in medical terms—I have called the ætiology of the conversion process. Since in unexpected and fulminant conversion the declaration of the immediate cause is always emphasized, the convert believes that ' grace ' is manifested in the determining cause, no matter what sort it may be ; a vision, or a trauma, an exceptional circumstance, or even an ordinary occurrence.

CHAPTER III

TYPES OF CONVERSION

A LL writers, whether they be historians or psychologists, divide conversion into two categories:
the fulminant or lightning type, and the progressive
type. If I am not mistaken, Starbuck's classification
of conversion into the impulsive and the volitional
types is a mere paraphrasing of the classic division.
I may state that from my own direct personal observation
and critical reflection I would regard such a division
as applicable only to the *duration* (rapid or slow) of the
conversional process. As to the *manner* of the conversion, there is only one. But let us proceed more
slowly.

1. *Conversion : Fulminant and Progressive :*
The Unconscious

All writers are agreed that fulminant, or lightning
conversions occur for the most part in connection with
some important or trivial event of the external or internal
life : a plastic vision, voices, a luminous nocturnal
phenomenon, or some other less significant circumstance.
The subject testifies to having experienced a sudden
overturning of his whole being ; the entire course of his
life is changed. St. Paul is the classic example of the
lightning type of conversion. Also the old religious
books describe all religious conversions in the same way
as they describe ' cures ' miraculously effected at the
touch of the magician, the rabbi, or the saint. It is not,

then, without significance, that books which deal with modern conversions tend rather to consider conversion as a psychical process, quite capable of analysis. Kurt Rothe [1] and Georges Valois [2] provide examples.

It must here be clearly understood that psychical regeneration may take place instantaneously; and this not merely in those who appeal to the 'grace' of the Christians, as when Dante, likening himself to the mystic Glaucus of Ovid's *Metamorphoses*, prepared his soul for the contemplation of the mysteries of Paradise; but also in those persons who appeal to history and to science. A sudden mystical experience has often led an individual to a transfiguration or trans-humanization; in short, to a renewal of the spirit. The ecstasies of the initiates into the Eleusinian mysteries were nothing other than a liberation, a catharsis, a regeneration of the soul.

In our inquiry, however, we are not considering possibilities, but actual occurrences. We are concerned simply to ascertain whether the fulminant type of religious conversion occurs, and if so, how often.

We are struck with the curious fact that the interpretation of certain conversions as instantaneous and perfectly passive, is maintained with no little heat both by the positivist psychologists and by those theologians who display the utmost jealousy for the prerogatives of 'grace'. Leuba,[3] for example, says that the moment of the actual conversion is turbulent, violent, rapid, passive, that is to say, involuntary and instantaneous. Silence, the night, bodily immobility—these are its frequent conditions. The concomitance of auditions, of luminous phenomena, of diverse physical sensations— especially of the muscular sense — is of frequent occurrence. And invariably there results a sense of relief, of liberation, even of joy, and at times, of the most

ineffable tenderness and love. Here there is no difference
between the interpretation of Leuba and the interpretation
of Father Mainage, except that with Leuba the operator
is chance, while with Mainage it is Christ.[4] But with
neither of these writers does the operator appear to be
the individual convert himself, excepting in so far as
Mainage, in accordance with the theological doctrine,
admits that the convert may have co-operated previously,
in the sense of having ' merited ' the consolatory crisis.

The agreement between two such opposed schools of
thought, and in particular the widespread approval of
the view of Leuba and many other psychologists concerning the interpretation of fulminant conversion, was
to be anticipated on account of the great developments
which have occurred of recent years in the study of .the
unconscious.   This study was formerly almost entirely
restricted to the domain of psychiatry, but has invaded
almost the whole field of psychology in consequence
of the researches of James, Myers [5], and Freud.[6] In
reality, even before this development of the study of
the unconscious occurred, the genetic method had led
physicians and psychologists to search in the biographies
of converts for the anticipatory indications of their mutation.   And this sort of investigation proved so fruitful
that the theologians learned to consider these antecedent
experiences the conscious preparation for receiving
' grace'. But then the unconscious intervened.

I do not here intend to rehearse to the reader what he
can find in so many books and memoirs, but I must not
shirk the duty of elaborating my point of view in regard
to this particular problem, where the theory of the
unconscious appears to dominate in an almost triumphal
fashion.

It must be recognized that two extreme psychological theories have been definitely abandoned: that of the Cartesians and of the Scottish school, who considered the psychical simply as the conscious; and on the other hand, Maudsley's theory of consciousness as epiphenomenal. In reality, a psychic sphere beyond the margins of consciousness does exist. Modern psychology has rightly readopted the traditions of St. Augustine and Leibnitz. The conception of psychological latency has now become of such fundamental importance that it serves to explain all psychic activity. Every psychologist recognizes the so-called 'implicit' representations, 'mediated' association, the formation of representative and conceptual groupings, intuition, and so forth. Ach, Marbe, Bühler, and others have demonstrated the importance of unconscious processes in the formation of concepts, conclusions, and determinations. One might here recall the phrase with which Ribot [7] concludes his book: " La psychologie de l'abstraction est en grande partie une psychologie de l'inconscient ", which means that a great part of synthetic activity has its roots in the unconscious.

We must, however, first state clearly what we mean by the term *unconscious*. The metaphysical unconscious does not concern us here. Equally, if by unconscious is meant something extrapersonal, that is, existing outside of man and attributable, for instance, to the processes of nature, this does not come within the purview of psychology. Nor, in our opinion, can an unconscious such as the *subliminal* of Myers, which has an autonomous existence with its own finality, as if there were a personality hidden within us operating without reference to conscious reality, be considered as within the ambit of scientific psychology. We cannot, in short, subscribe to the doctrine of the

omnipotent subliminal, according to which the greater
and truer Ego hidden in every man may display itself
suddenly, like an insurgent will, eluding the vigilance of
consciousness, even overwhelming it, only allowing it to
survive in order to confess its own subordination. Here
we are in the field of interpretation of fact; at most the
Myers theory may be taken as a mere hypothesis if it be
shorn of all its superstructure, as in Myers's presentation.

It must be confessed that the hypothesis of the
subliminal is exceedingly useful for clarifying the interpretation of the interminable series of facts which make up
so-called ' supernormal ' psychology.   But it is probably
more profitable to collect, criticize, and classify the facts
than to indulge in the discussion of hypotheses which
are attractive, perhaps, but for that very reason must
not be too readily accepted as principles.

For us it appears an absolute certainty that the
unconscious is in continuous connection with the conscious,
and actually is not as independent of it as some would
have us believe.[8]   On this point we are certainly in
agreement with Jastrow,[9] who controverts the theories
of Myers.   Nevertheless, in oneiric activity one may
recognize this claim to independence.

The conscious psyche is the fulfilment and the perfection
of the subconscious, since it not only represents a
' selection ' from the psychic mass, but also intensifies,
defines—one might almost say individualizes—the
psychic content.   Our social adaptation is made up of
new or quasi-improvised acts; it is composed of
syntheses, or of new combinations of old acts.   But
adaptation, improvisation, and combination are the
work of consciousness.   Thus it is that consciousness
displays itself as a unifying activity, though variable
in its contents and in its levels or grades (according to

Westphall).   With Leibnitz and many others, we would maintain that true volitions belong to the conscious sphere, and not to the unconscious, in which we can only discover ' tendencies to volitions ' or ' reproductions of past volitions ', and not true, complete, or original volitions.

Moreover, we cannot be sure that true judgment and reasoning exist in the unconscious. They may seem to occur, for instance unconscious reasoning seems to occur in perceptions and illusions. But in reality these are rather ' habits of decision ' than true ratiocinations, or else they are the repetitions (in response to certain stimuli) of former dynamic cerebral states, that is, *unconscious returns* of past judgments and reasonings which were *formerly conscious*. In short, the volitions and the thoughts of the unconscious, like the images and the feelings which have resulted from past experiences, are dispositions which return to actuality ; they are not original formations. Whatever original matter may be discovered in recollection—and this occurs invariably, even in the most ' faithful ' recollections— can be traced ultimately to the actual moment in which the recollection is formed in the consciousness.

That the whole unconscious mass is capable of organizing itself into a sort of subconscious or co-conscious personality, as Morton Prince has put it,[10] can be accepted without difficulty. But that is an ephemeral occurrence in which is involved, much more than is supposed, the primary consciousness of the subject who is under hypnotic influence, or who has become ' depersonalized '.

Certain exceptional states of the psyche in which the unconscious experience is uppermost are undoubtedly of great interest : such are dreams, *rêveries*, æsthetic contemplation, ecstasies, ravishments, dual personalities, syncopes, anguish. But none of these exceptional conditions can legitimately be exalted above the normal state of full consciousness. It is of the greatest psychological interest to explore the marginal regions of the consciousness, either spontaneously, or by scientific experiment, or through æsthetic or mystical exaltation, and so to obtain a rapid experience of the non-differentiated thought of primitive man or of childhood, which is free from all the trammels of logic and of representation. But those who exalt the exceptional beyond the normal—over-estimating the content of such exceptional experience, and deducing therefrom doctrines of a philosophical or moral nature—merely condemn the conscious to a subjection to the unconscious. But man is possessed of normal aspiration towards the conscious, the decisive, the definite, which implies an aspiration towards group life and towards human solidarity.

The object of child-education, in fact, is to make the child conscious ; to give plastic form to his thoughts, in order that he may understand and objectivate the world and himself by symbolic images. The pre-conscious psychic activity of the young child is only energy which awaits effective experience in order to become conscious ; which awaits the moment when it can assume its vestment, and become communicable and social. The upward movement for man is, then, towards the conscious and the rational. The downward movement is towards the subconscious, that is to say, down towards the dream, the blind enthusiasm, the unconditional abandon of the self.

In order to avoid misunderstanding we must formulate our thesis more precisely. In our own school of psychology, the significance of the term *subconscious* has, for many years, been clearly defined, in contradistinction to the term *unconscious*. This latter term has been specially reserved to signifiy such processes (e.g. physiological) as can never rise into the light of consciousness.

But in our ' subconscious ', on the other hand, are included the psychic ' minims ', that is, psychic night and twilight ; the passive reverie ; the dream-state ; the ' active reverie ' of Beaunis ; the marginal and the extra-marginal consciousness of James ; the ' minimal ' or infinitesimal consciousness of Aliotta ; the pathological psychic automatism of Janet and the alienists ; and a part, too, of the unconscious (*Unbewusste*) of Freud and his *Vorbewusste*, or ' preconscious '.

When in the present work it becomes necessary for me to employ the word unconscious, the reader will understand the meaning which I attach to the term.

Now comes the question : what are the contents of the subconscious as it is generally considered ? The structure of the subconscious results from perceptions (in the sense of Leibnitz), sentiments, images, ideas, judgments, ratiocinations, and finally, volitions. This is the view of many psychologists since Wundt (who made a masterly analysis of the subconscious), although they have exaggerated and somewhat deformed his thought.[11]

Admitting, for the moment, that the subconscious latent ' sphere ', or the ' opposite sphere ' as it is also termed, possesses this complex structure, we must inquire *in what form* do ideas, perceptions, feelings, and so forth exist there ?

D'Annunzio has written : " Actions lie asleep in a race like the fœtus curled up within its mother's womb."

This is well enough as literature ; but such metaphors belong to poetry rather than to the scientific spirit. Often the answer to the question of what is meant by memory or latent thought is a reference to the two theories already applied to representation : the *Substanztheorie* or the *Aktualitätstheorie*. According to the latter theory—which does not contradict the doctrine of cortical localization, but rather corrects and interprets it — these terms mean dispositions, capacities for receiving impressions (as John Stuart Mill says) ; not potential dispositions, but dispositions which become realized, once the way is clear ; dynamic tendencies, in short. This is the point of view which we accept. For us the dynamic force of the subconscious or the ' latent sphere ' is a certainty. The old philosophic conception of intellectual habits appears to us to be manifestly inadequate.

Modern psychology explains these ' dispositions ' by means of the concept of Activity, or of a psychic *en*, thereby recognizing merely their physiological aspect as states of potential nervous energy. This, of course, it is not our purpose to explain. For the purpose of our inquiry it may, however, be taken for granted that the subconscious contents cannot be described simply as organic conditions, but, according to our parallelistic hypothesis, are physico-chemical conditions associated with psychic energy, or to express it differently, they are ' psycho-physical tendencies '. The unconscious, however, is *strictiori sensu* exclusively organic.

Ribot [12] maintains that a kinæsthetic element is present in every intellectual process. Every association, he declares, is an association of movements ; motor activity interpenetrates the whole of psychic existence. According to Ribot's hypothesis, therefore, the subconscious would consist of the kinæsthetic portion of conscious states ; motor phenomena which, to a greater extent than all others, possess the tendency towards organization and solidification. All this can be admitted. The experimental psychology of sensation, or of imagination, or of attention, confirms the existence of a motor element in states of consciousness, either with or without external realization.

In fact one may take it as proven that every thought has its motor side ; that there is nothing psychic without some sort of correlative ' behaviour '. The so-called motor vibrations of thought have in fact been discovered by experimental psychology in the vascular system, in the glands, in the phonetic muscles, in those of the fingers, etc. It must also be added that mental pathology discloses motor elements in morbid phenomena, deriving from the most profound depths of the subconscious. But this theory of Ribot's would seem to be incomplete unless one adds that these kinæsthetic elements preserve in all of us a species of ' record ' of those contents to which they were once joined. This implies a particular kind of disposition and orientation. And if this be so they can only be regarded as ' differentiated ', not generic, kinæsthetic elements.

In conclusion, then, we find ourselves able to assert— for the purpose of a clearer orientation—that the subconscious is made up of ' dispositions ' or tendencies, complete and dynamic, which may be conceived of as a sort of animated mould, ready to receive contents ; but with this peculiarity : that each mould is specially adapted for the reception of some particular kind of content, and no other.

It is difficult to admit pre-formed images, ideas, or movements ; that is to say, elements already thrown into moulds and transmitted just as they are by heredity. There are, however, certain facts which might make us suspect this. At least we can safeguard ourselves in so audacious an hypothesis by imparting to the 'dispositions' the sense already given, which is precisely that which modern psychology assigns to the mnemonic 'paths'. The matter which is to be cast into these dynamic moulds—a certain given matter and no other— or matter attracted by the mould towards itself, is material which, more frequently than is imagined, is supplied by the experiences of consciousness.

One may consider the subconscious mass as being in a state of tension, in comparison with the conscious actuality, which can be considered as energy in action. Otherwise, the actual *en* of the conscious could not constitute the exact antithesis of the potential *en* of the subconscious. The subconscious content does not explode at intervals, but in reality operates in a continuous, albeit inconspicuous, manner. This is demonstrated by innumerable facts of ordinary daily life. It suffices to remember that our most secret tendencies, aspirations, and passions, unsuspected by us, betray themselves continually in gestures, in set phrases, in *lapsus* [13], in wit, in the play of associations, and especially in spontaneous free associations.

What stimuli determine the great explosions and the small continual psycho-energetic escapes of subconscious experiences ? This is a difficult question, requiring to be answered with some breadth. An enumeration must here suffice. The 'dispositional mass' is realized in thoughts, sentiments, motions, and actions by reflex dynamogeny, not (in spite of what the physiologists say) by automatism. Therefore the combined psychic reflexes work harmoniously and as one in both the

conscious and the subconscious spheres. Very rarely
they exhaust themselves in one of the two spheres,
but may be said to pervade them both. Thus it is that
the ordinary stimuli provocative of subconscious realizations almost always derive from conscious reality. There
are conscious-unconscious reflexes, since in the first phase
they may be conscious. This is one instance of that
close relationship, which we have already admitted,
between the two facets of psychic activity. It may
happen, however, that the realizations of the subconscious are self-initiated ; the psychic reflex, in that
case, is unconscious, at least in its first and second
phases of manifestation. It is only in the third phase—
that of motion—that it becomes perceptible. Subsequent reflection, hypnosis, or psycho-analysis may
reconstruct the topography of such reflexes, but generally
they escape superficial analysis. The third phase—
being conscious—offers us a guiding thread which
leads to the discovery of the primary or original
phase.

To facilitate inquiry and interpretation we must cease
to think of the 'subconscious mass' or of the
'dispositional psyche', as an accumulation of contents
preserved in a random fashion. There are curious
phenomena and rigorously logical deductions which lead
us to imagine the mass as stratified, like the layers
forming the crust of the earth, which have been deposited
at different levels corresponding with the period of their
formation. Janet has already compared the subconscious with geological strata. We can, indeed,
devise a diagram of such a stratification, proceeding from below upwards, in brief outline, as
follows :—

I. The hereditary or pre-formed unconscious.
- (a) Of the species (instincts).
- (b) Racial.
- (c) Historical or Ethnic.
- (d) Family.

II. The unconscious of the developmental periods.
- (a) Ante-natal.
- (b) Of early Infancy.
- (c) Of late Infancy.
- (d) Of Childhood and Adolescence.

III. The late unconscious of the post-developmental period.
- (a) Of Adult life.
- (b) Experience of Life and Culture.[14]

This is no mere fantasy. In the actual life of every day, in hypnosis, in mental pathology, and even in dreams, striking proofs are to be found of this stratification of the imaginal and affective-volitional dispositions. At times the stratification of the memory appears clearly ; particularly in cases of aphasia and of the grosser lesions of the brain.

Recapitulating, then, we may postulate that psychic activity is the result of the setting in action of the two dynamic masses : actual and latent. The *actual mass* is dynamic in accordance with the impulses which it receives from the necessity of new adaptations to the environment, or from the will. The *latent mass* is dynamic in accordance with the impulses which it receives from older adaptations. The dynamogeny which moves the latent mass forces it into contact with the actual mass ; producing either a ' conflict ' or an accord between the two. In fact, as everyone realizes, we can live in our old adaptations ; that is to say, in the instincts, the tendencies, the habits, in all the ' pre-volitional ' experiences ; or we can live in conflict with them, opposing to them efforts towards new adaptations. There is in short *accord* in reflex, instinctive, and automatic activity ; and *conflict* in volitional activity, which tends to develop fresh situations from those already experienced. In sleep the accord is complete, at least in profound sleep ; it is incomplete when sleep is light and its curve oscillates considerably so that consciousness is not completely submerged. Many painful dreams are directly due to conflicts between the subconscious and the conscious reality, which is not completely inactive even during sleep.[15]

2. *The Fulminant Type of Conversion*

Returning, now, to our theme, we find that William James regarded instantaneous conversion as the true type ;[16] and, indeed, this is supported by the testimony of many converts. It is, however, probable that James, who adhered over-fixedly to his interpretation (Myers's theory of the sublimal) has somewhat exaggerated, or has somewhat unduly extended, the conception of instantaneity. It is certain that when we attempt to probe deeper in our study of sudden converts, we discover that the *coup de foudre*, which in the main is observable in only a small minority of conversions, is in fact the least significant, though the most æsthetic, moment of the conversion.

In any case, it is not the event itself, but rather the conscious reflection that immediately follows, which determines the change, that is, the conversion, properly so called. These reflections are rarely instantaneous and are much less so in those cases in which the resistance of the will has to be overcome. The *coup de foudre* would appear to constitute the pivot of the conversion ; but in actual fact it is either the point of departure or the point of arrival.

F

If I am not mistaken, conversion is frequently confused with other psychic processes : for instance with invention, or faith, or inspiration. Quite different, however, are the dynamics of invention, and of the different intellectual processes in general. In these, indeed, the suddenness may be evident, and the action of the subconscious extremely rapid and decisive. The mathematician, Henri Poincaré, for instance, in one of his lectures, has related how he had suddenly seen revealed the solution of a problem in mathematics upon which he had been working for two years. The revelation came at the moment when he was called up for military service during the recent war, and was entering the train with a number of companions. Having reached the solution, the inventor developed it and applied it in the light of consciousness, but his personality did not undergo, on this account, the least mutation. Conversion is something entirely different.

Inspiration is an illumination which clarifies a truth already perceived, or reveals a new truth. Prophetic inspiration is all this, and it is, according to Delacroix, also the sense of having a mission. In any case, inspiration, as Nietzsche observed in himself, is a whirlwind which sweeps on, and in which individual liberty has no part. The divine inspiration is ' grace ' ; it is the ' gift of God ', and is therefore beyond the control of the subject.

Mozart said he knew nothing of his art, because he did not enter into it. Ruskin once wrote to Rossetti that one thing of which he was sure in this world was that the very best work that a man does, is done without effort ; that immediate effort produces an imperfect work.

We do not know of any convert in history who has said as much. In spite of the most explicit recognition of ' grace ', all the converted speak of their crises, of their efforts, and of the conflicts which they have endured. This means that the subconscious material reached the consciousness of the subject unelaborated, and that he had not only to hold it strongly in check, but to elaborate it by connecting it with strong· links to the whole of his experience.

Similarly, many people confuse the emotion of faith with conversion. Conversion, most emphatically, must not be identified with belief. Faith as a religious experience or as a mystic intuition of the divine is only a moment of the conversion. Luciano Puel de Lobel, one of the converts whose experiences are given in Mainage's collection, describes the intuition of the divine as " an interior audition of mystic music, rich with living and profound joy, and resulting from a perfect momentary harmony effected between the subconscious and the Mysterious Beyond ". A ' momentary ' unification, this, while conversion is a stable and lasting condition of the consciousness.

It is hardly permissible to hold that in the case of ' lightning ' conversion the consciousness of the subject has never experienced, prior to the crisis, the beginnings of mutation, that is, displacement of the " habitual centre of personal energy ", to use William James's expression. For the catechumen to the faith, the sense of disgust, or at the least of distaste, for his old pleasures and his old habits ; his doubts concerning whether he is on the right track ; his longings for solitude ; his need for a fixed aim and for the equilibrium of his conscience—all these are the conscious preliminary symptoms of conversion, however little conversion is invested with the splendour of reality in his prevision. He is already listening to the voice which calls to him from afar, but he

is unable thoroughly to understand its meaning, because
he is constantly disturbed by the tempest of the soul.
The psychiatrist, Rogues De Fursac, justly observes that
a fleeting remorse, an aspiration towards better things,
had often been noticed among the antecedent phenomena
of the Welsh alcoholic converts.

If we check our enthusiasm for the unconscious,
we may investigate the 'conscious' antecedents of
religious mutations with greater profit, and then perhaps
the discontinuous but constant relations between the
conscious and the unconscious will be better recognized.

Even the non-theological criticism of facts in connection with instantaneity appears to me to be of distinct
value. St. Paul, scribe and Pharisee, and persecutor of
the Nazarenes, but (at any rate according to the German
theologians) in contact with the Hellenistic world of
Tarsus in Cilicia, was agitated by doubts, even before
the vision on the dusty, sun-parched road to Damascus.
His conversion, then, may not have been instantaneous.
In truth, very little is actually known of the conversion
of St. Paul.[17] Probably his eyes were blinded by the
heat and the glare ; we have no way of knowing if the
attack was epileptic. Renan does not speak of epilepsy,
though he is prodigal in medical explanations, such as
pernicious fever, sunstroke, brain-storm, or a thunderbolt.
It is curious that the chief witness to the fact is
St. Paul himself—the unconscious, the epileptic. He it
is who recounts the words which were spoken to him by
Jesus in the Syriac-Aramaic language, while the texts
are not in perfect agreement among themselves in their
accounts of the testimony of the other witnesses who
were present.

It is true that St. Paul speaks of his conversion as
being absolutely unforeseen, and we possess no reliable

documents by which to contradict him. At any rate
one may hold, without doing violence to the accounts
in Acts, that the vivid impressions which Paul carried
away of the vision, followed by the fever and the
blindness, when " he was three days without sight ",
were the occasion of profound reflection ; and that his
conversion—like his decision to preach in Damascus,
and to proceed to Jerusalem, where he would meet the
disciples of Jesus—was the fruit of that conscious
reflection and not of the moment of his vision. This,
however, in no way contradicts the statement of St. Paul,
that no human instrument intervened in his conversion.

Everyone will recall the famous scene of St. Augustine
in the garden.[18] One day, in a mood of extreme
uneasiness, he spoke to Alypius in an exalted fashion,
and feeling a desire to weep in solitude he went into the
garden. Alypius, deeply moved, followed him, but
Augustine took no notice of him. His heart was in agony.
He loathed himself for his sins and for his vileness.
Suddenly he arose, ran to a fig tree, and, throwing himself
on the ground, burst into sobs. It was at this moment
that the voice of a child in a neighbouring house began
to repeat in cadence the words : *Tolle et lege.* Augustine
started in surprise ; it was a divine command. He
went back again to the spot where Alypius was and
where he had left the Epistles of St. Paul. He opened
the book and read. His anguish had ceased. He had
regained tranquillity.

Who could believe that it was precisely at the instant
of *tolle et lege* that the transformation of St. Augustine
was initiated ? Some would have us believe that the
initiation of his conversion should date from the reading
of Cicero's *Hortensius*, when he was nineteen ; others
say that it must have been during his sojourn in Rome ;

others, again, during the time he spent in Milan, listening
to discourses of St. Ambrose. But, whenever it happened,
what St. Augustine writes in his *Confessions* is of much
importance. " I declare unto you that it was as one
walking who turns backward, and looks toward religion,
which is in us children, as is the marrow within the bones
of our forefathers. Or to state this better : it was
without my own doing that I was drawn thitherwards.
Through hesitation, and in haste and uncertainty, I took
up the writings of Paul, and with supreme attention and
prudence I read them from beginning to end." [19] From
this it is clear that in connection with St. Augustine's
conversion one cannot apply the word instantaneous.

Concerning the conversion of St. Francis of Assisi
the authorities are not all in agreement, but about the
following particulars there seems to be little doubt.[20]
In the year 1202 St. Francis was imprisoned at Perugia,
where he remained a year. On his release, at about the
age of twenty-one, he was suffering from a grave malady
which weakened him considerably. It was at this
particular period that he became conscious in his soul
of the vanity of all things and of the emptiness of the
world. " He began to grow small in his own eyes ",
as his biographer, Tomaso Celano, puts it. It was then
that he developed his ardent love for the poor. After
some time he had his famous ' dream of the palace ',
which caused him to reflect on his vocation. St. Francis,
by slow degrees, began to understand clearly that it was
his destiny to accomplish great and decisive things.
While he was in Assisi, preparations for the expedition
to Apulia, under the command of Walter III, were being
made. St. Francis, desirous of military glory, decided to
enroll. It seems that the night before his departure for
Spoleto, he had a dream which influenced his decision

to fight. But at Spoleto he probably had a fever, at all events it is certain that he heard an admonitory voice dissuading him from military life. In fact, that very day he retraced his way to Assisi. Interior conflicts were manifested in St. Francis's uncertain behaviour. In Assisi he resumed his life of gaiety, while, at the same time, his mutation was progressing. At this period prayer and his ardent love of poverty took a great part in his conscious life. One cannot say, however, that his conversion was matured or completed before 1205, when he made a pilgrimage to Rome to visit the tombs of the apostles.

The famous *Thurmerlebnis* of Luther is given great importance in his separation from the Church of Rome.[21] It cannot be denied that in 1514 Luther, when undergoing this ' experience of the tower ', became aware of the illuminating significance of the *Justitia Dei* of St. Paul's Epistle to the Romans, and may have had the sensation of the ' good tidings ' contained in the Gospel ; but this experience was certainly not the *coup de foudre* which determined his separation. This separation was a long and laborious process, which lasted from 1510 until 1515 and which included serious intellectual and affective crises and the celebrated ' Consolations '.

We next turn to the consideration of some modern cases. It is related that the conversion of the Italian novelist, Manzoni, occurred while gazing at a Madonna in one of the churches in Paris ; but this is only a legend. It is well known from his biographers how, for some time before his conversion, the great writer deeply grieved over his defects and his sins, and tried to find the way to a better life. It was towards the end of 1808, still before the conversion of his wife, that he had his first-born child baptized with the rites of the Catholic faith.

The process of Manzoni's religious mutation lasted over several years. He felt a decisive impulse in 1810, when his wife, Enrichetta, passed over from Protestantism to Catholicism. But his own conversion was not completed until 1811.[22]

Again, it has been believed that the conversion of Cardinal Newman was the result of the reading of an article by Cardinal Wiseman in the *Dublin Review* ; or resulted from the perception of a new meaning in the words of St. Augustine : " *securas judicat orbis terrarum.*" [23] But the story of the interior conflicts of this great soul is in open contradiction to this fable. When Newman, on 9th October, 1845, placed his abjuration in the hands of Father Dominic, the Passionist, he only completed an act which had become imperative to him after the progressive, slow, and conflicting mutation—outward and inward—which had begun before 1839, the year during which the famous 'Oxford Movement' had reached its height. The psychologist cannot avoid recalling how Newman, with his friend Hurrel Froude, came to Rome in 1832, and visited Cardinal Wiseman, then Rector of the English College. From Rome they went on to Sicily, and at Termini Imerese Newman fell gravely ill, and was then heard to say, in the delirium of his fever, as he himself records in his *Apologia* : " No, I cannot die, because I have not sinned against the light, which I have not yet seen." His disquietude and aspirations towards the light reveal the subconscious struggle leading towards his conversion, which, however, was slowly and consciously matured, through the Oxford Movement, and the publication of the *Tracts for the Times*.

It is certainly strange how almost all converts like to believe in the suddenness of their mutation. François

Coppée declared that his conversion was *soudaine*, though from his own story one can deduce, on the contrary, that his conversion was slow, and consciously slow. '*Soudaine*' it may perhaps have seemed to Coppée, because he was able to state definitely the day in October, 1897, when he was conscious of being sufficiently changed to receive the Communion.

Durtal, the hero in Huysmans's novel, *En Route*, also declared: "*soudain je crois*", and explained that he had been unaware of his mutation, just as one is unaware of his digestive processes. Yet Huysmans's entire novel is nothing but the story of the protracted conflicts of a soul desiring to become converted to the Catholic faith.

André de Bavier declared: "I do believe", on the morning of Easter, 1912, at the elevation of the consecrated Host. But to me it appears clear that this convert is confusing his mutation—which is a matter of practice—with certain moments of faith which are, indeed, necessary, but which do not alone suffice for the process of conversion.

Hermann Ronge (Johannes Jœrgensen) was converted from rationalism to Catholicism during the midnight Christmas mass in a church at Monaco, at the moment when the *Gloria in Excelsis* was chanted. It is enough to read the antecedents of Hermann Ronge's conversion to convince oneself that this mutation had been initiated some time before and that the process of his conversion was clearly perceptible to him.

The Polish philosopher Lutoslawski, as he related at the Congress of Geneva, experienced conversion while in the bath. This was, however, only the banal circumstance to which his memory referred the mutation, which to his own knowledge had been initiated long

before.   In fact at the age of sixteen, in 1879, he had had
a violent mental crisis, lasting several weeks, in which
he was tormented by doubts, and implored Christ to
manifest Himself to him, unequivocably and absolutely.[24]
He had obtained no clear sign and so rejected the faith
of his fathers.   After this, a bishop and others tried to
convert him.   He discussed religion with a younger
brother, who afterwards became a priest, and he made
a study of Dante and a commentary on his philosophy.
During the period subsequent to his dispute with the
Faculty of Philosophy of Cracow University—in which
Lutoslawski was successful and his self-esteem thereby
much increased—the episode of the bath occurred.
He had been taking a vapour bath, in which he had
thoroughly cleansed his body, when the idea came to
him to cleanse his soul as well, although he had no
particular cause for self-reproach.   However, he went
at once to a church and there made his confession to
a very ignorant Franciscan friar.   He even told the
confessor that he could not communicate, because he
did not believe in the real presence of Christ in the
Eucharist.   The Franciscan nevertheless bade him do so,
on his own responsibility.   And then, he said, there
occurred suddenly the essential fact which changed all
his life.   At the very moment of receiving communion,
he unexpectedly understood everything and above all
received an imperative command from an indisputable
power, to unite his life for ever with the Church which
he had abandoned twenty years before.   It was, in his
phrase, "like a flash of lightning, comparable to the
conversion of St. Paul ".

It seems clear to me that there was not, during the
bath of the Polish philosopher, any unforeseen and sudden
irruption of subconscious experiences, coming from the

ultra-marginal life, of which James, Morton Prince, and so many others speak with such assurance ; irruptions which are equivalent to the imposition of certainty and are the cause of a radical mutation in life.[25]

I may briefly summarize the process of conversion of another convert, with whom I obtained an interview in 1921. This subject had a religious upbringing, but he quickly became an atheist and an extremist in politics. He had always been a man of action, with keen interest in culture. During his youth, the problem of religion both interested and disquieted him. About his thirtieth year his religious preoccupation became a conscious anguish. One night in which his agony was most acute, he felt within him a sort of beneficent change, and he saw—always in his imagination—a kind of shining body, like a golden egg. Next day he felt tranquil and was able to recite one of the prayers of his childhood, learnt from his mother. For the last five years he has been a militant Catholic. Was this a fulminant conversion, determined by the ' egg of gold ' ? It might seem so from his own account ; but there was a preceding change of faith ; the modification of his life had been accomplished, little by little.

In autobiographical accounts we often find the expression ' an inner call '. We are dealing, here, with a form of inspiration, and can appreciate the tremendous persuasive power of such an experience. In the majority of cases it transpires, however, that before the call the subject was clearly conscious of his future destiny. It is, indeed, by no means rare for the law-maker, the prophet, or the saint to retire voluntarily into solitude and obscurity, expressly to hear—one might say *to solicit*—the inspiration or the call itself. The history of religion is filled with such instances, from Moses on

Sinai, and Jesus in the desert, to St. Ignatius in the Grotto of Manresa. Of the same description was the famous vision of Descartes, when he saw himself as the reformer of philosophy, which in reality was only the seal of his conscious programme.

Another example of the lightning type of conversion, cited by both James and Mainage, is that of the young French Jew who afterwards became Father Alphonse-Marie Ratisbonne.[26] He, too—as is usual—in his own account characterizes his conversion as instantaneous.

On the 20th January, 1842, he went into the church of Sant' Andrea delle Fratte, in Rome, where for a few moments he was entirely alone. Suddenly he experienced an unforeseen and profound inner mutation ; it was like a man who was born blind, at one flash seeing the light. Before proceeding to the interpretation which Ratisbonne himself has given of his conversion, one must turn to the facts in a disinterested spirit. And they are these.

Alphonse Charles Tobias Ratisbonne was born in a Jewish family at Strasbourg in 1814. He has stated that at about the age of fourteen or fifteen he studied the Hebrew religion ; from this time until the age of twenty-three he had no religion, " not even a belief in God ". In consequence of his love for his Jewish niece, he turned to devotion for the Hebrew religion, and at the same time to a hatred of Christianity and of his brother Theodore, who was already a convert to Christianity and a priest. In his youth Ratisbonne had read the story of Theodore's conversion, and had skimmed the pages of a life of St. Bernard, written by his brother. He had also read some pages of a book on Christian doctrine by Lhomond. At the age of twenty-eight he came to Rome, on a pleasure trip. There he met Baron Theodore de Bussières. a convert from Calvinism to Catholicism.

and an intimate friend of his brother's. He visited the church of Ara Cœli, receiving "a profoundly moving impression". One day he saw de Bussières, who gave him a medal with the image of the Virgin and, out of politeness, he allowed it to be hung round his neck, He further accepted from de Bussières a prayer of St. Bernard, the *Memorare*, and he promised to recite it. Ratisbonne transcribed the prayer and, in reading it, learnt it by heart. " It impressed itself on my spirit and I could not avoid repeating it to myself." From the 16th of January to the date of his conversion Ratisbonne was constantly in the company of de Bussières, and under his influence. They visited churches and Christian monuments together. Ratisbonne confesses that he felt even then a repugnance and scorn for Catholicism. The biographer, however, records that " Ratisbonne, however much he attempted to dissimulate it, was disturbed ". During the night between the 19th and 20th of January he was aroused and saw a great dark cross ; and no matter how much he tried to dismiss this vision, he saw it constantly before his eyes, so that he could not sleep. On the 20th of January he went with de Bussières to Sant' Andrea delle Fratte, for a funeral. It chanced that he remained in the church alone for a moment, and it was then that he felt and " saw something like a veil before him and in the centre of the dimness the image of the Virgin ", with the same attitude and appearance as that of the miraculous medal of the Immaculate Conception. " At this vision I fell upon my knees . . . I knew the horror of my state . . . and the beauty of the Catholic religion: in one word, I understood all." To his interrogators Ratisbonne declared : " I cannot explain such a mutation unless I compare it to that of a man suddenly awakened from a deep sleep, or to that of a man, born blind, who has received sight at one stroke."

Let us, at the outset, observe that these details are autobiographical notes, and therefore susceptible of every criticism. The good faith of Ratisbonne is unquestionable, but it is legitimate to suppose that, after his conversion, his principal—indeed one might almost say his sole—preoccupation was to give the greatest possible value to the circumstances of his conversion, *ad majorem Dei gloriam*, and for the edification of the faithful. Nevertheless Ratisbonne himself informs us: *firstly*, that he loved and he hated; he therefore manifested in himself that richness of emotion which is one of the predisposing factors in profound mutations; *secondly*, that Christianity, Catholicism, conversions, and even books of devotion were known to his consciousness; *thirdly*, that in Rome he had had a long intimacy with the devoutly Catholic de Bussières, with whom he had visited churches; *fourthly*, that he had accepted the famous medal, which he, in full consciousness, wore round his neck, and St. Bernard's prayer, which he repeated and got by heart; *fifthly*, that in these days he was continually putting the question of conversion to himself, and always decided by a negative; the dissimulation of the conflict is a sure proof of this. However, the case of Ratisbonne came to be considered as exceptional, even by those who quote it as a typical example of fulminant conversion. It has not seemed superfluous, therefore, to probe rather deeply the motives of such an exceptional case.

I think that it is in no way derogatory to converts to suppose that they, urged by the desire to enhance the workings of 'grace', and influenced by apologetic aims, may involuntarily curtail in their accounts the conscious antecedents of their mutations. One may conclude that the so-called unconsciousness of conversion does not always refer to the actual event, but to the moment of its description; so that the circumstances should not be termed *unconscious*, but *forgotten*; the amnesia (in these cases being, in a varying degree, justified) completely blots out the conscious phases of the process, at the moment of the testimony. A 'strong state of the soul'—whether taking the form of an image as vivid as hallucination, a stinging desire, an intense emotion (as, for example, an occurrence in the War)—can blur and falsify the memory. Of this centuries-old psycho-physical truth mythology has possessed itself, crystallized in the famous draught, or philtre, of oblivion. Wagner, for example, avails himself of this myth in *Siegfried*, who when passion for Gudrun seizes him, forgets Brunhilde after drinking the narcotic which Hagen offers him. Mythology apart, however, it is certainly widely accepted, both in psychology and in mental pathology, that undergoing an emotional shock or witnessing any prodigious or solemn spectacle suffices to blot out, to blur, to render imperceptible, or in some such manner to destroy the mnemonic pictures nearest in time and space to the occurrence itself.

It must be noted, however, that this forgetfulness does not therefore imply a pathological character in conversion; since the formation of a *sense of novelty*, like its abolition—paramnesia—is now explained by psychologists as a peculiar state of the subject's consciousness, and not as pathological.

The same phenomenon may occur in certain exceptional cases, in which the apparent starting-point of the conversion becomes fixed specifically in a vision, a trauma,

or a profound grief. The shock acts as the philtre ;
and the convert, in all good faith, may forget his
antecedent mutations, or, at any rate, find the memory
of them negligible in his consciousness.

In one of its phases conversion is assuredly subconscious. There is, of course, as we have already
stated, a subconscious phase in all psychological processes.
The psychologist recognizes psychic moments still more
interesting, which might seem to explain the conversion,
and yet do not in any way explain it. It happens,
occasionally, that a chance phrase, a word, a picture,
a person, an event, or a ceremony, seen and heard before
on countless occasions, suddenly assumes a new aspect
and is endowed with a meaning which it never had before.
Gratry, in his *Pages choisies*, alludes to this transformation
of words. There often occur intuitions, or rapid illumina-
tions, in individuals of superior intelligence or extreme
sensitiveness, and they may occur even to ordinary
people in exceptional moments. Many of us have
doubtless had this experience.

In certain individuals, then, and at certain solemn
moments in the life of the soul, there undoubtedly blaze
forth unforeseen spiritual flashes of inspiration ;
significant states of consciousness. The problem, nevertheless, remains : whether we can concede that the
dynamics of internal intuition (as exemplified in the
states of desire, hope, or æsthetic vision) can be identified
with the conversion itself. This identification cannot,
in my opinion, be sustained. To change oneself is not
the same as to believe ; illumination is not a practical
regeneration.

In the æsthetics of Croce, it is true, intuition is
identified with the internal expression ; and the work

of art is complete at that moment. But I do not feel able to subscribe to this doctrine of our celebrated philosopher. Without realization the work of art cannot be complete ; it is non-existent. The word, the concrete fact, is lacking. The greatest artists are able powerfully to realize their dreams. Art, morality, conversion—these consist in objective realization, and not in an intuitive possibility. In a few words : conversion starts from an intuition, as does every sort of psychic experience ; but it becomes complete only as a process, as conduct ; the value of the conversion is therefore entirely practical, otherwise it would be pure thought, not conversion.

Nor is the establishing of this fact without importance, in that the continuity of the conversion—which means the actual conversion itself—is conditioned by its practical realization. If it be true that *fides sine operibus mortua est*, with how much more reason can we say that conversion without conduct is no conversion. The realization is not a dead phase of the process ; it has a specific task : to animate the new experiences of religion. And it is on this account that the initial intuition remains vivifying and productive.[27]

One day some Parisian priests went into the forest to visit the great mystic Ruysbroeck, who instead of satisfying the curiosity of his visitors told them : " You are saints according to the measure of your desire to be such." The same can be said of conversion. The unforeseen, unexpected flashes of intuition are insufficient to produce lasting effects upon the consciousness, unless it has been adapted by preparation and unless it assumes a decisive attitude of action. In the same way, one cannot regard as either serious or lasting the philosophical and theological intuitions professed by many famous physicists and biologists during midnight seances in the presence of the phantoms evoked by Eusapia Paladino. Before the dawn of the next day every impression of the compromising exclamations they uttered the night before would have completely faded from their recollections.

The latent mass is constantly operating in us. To use the current expression: the unconscious is dynamic. What wonder then, that new and significant religious experience should suddenly or unexpectedly appear in consciousness with the rapidity and vividness due to the impulsion of such dynamic energy? Such cases might almost be termed common. They are normal, in fact, even outside the sphere of religion and mysticism. We suddenly realize the meaning of facts or of words as if it came to us from afar. A sudden volitional decision is as unforeseen as an explosion, and when it occurs we have the sense that it bursts forth from the periphery of the reflections on which we are engaged.

In conversion, however, we have something besides this, and something which is essential. The true conversional process begins, if ever, with the consciousness of these apparitions and experiences, and runs its full course by retaining these apparitions and experiences in the consciousness and definitely accepting them by the will. A conversion may certainly appear sudden and fulminant; but upon serious reflection it will be evident that the suddenness—if any—is only the perception of the significance, the realization of one's destiny, belief. All these are facts which, if sudden, are also by their very nature transitory, when the will to perceive, to understand, and to believe does not arrest them in their rapid flight.

It need scarcely surprise us to find a little water diluting the generous wine of the theory of the unconscious. The economy even of philosophy and science changes with time. To-day, if I am not mistaken, in spite of the fame and success of Freudianism, the theory is gradually undergoing a revision among psychologists. Once they were too ready to believe, for example, in the unconscious collaboration of races and multitudes in the formation of myths and legends. So to-day, by way of reaction, they are singling out the conscious creative individuals from the anonymous and ignorant masses. The same thing happens in the field of religious phenomena. Through full investigation it is possible to recognize the creative process in conscious construction or in renewal of the individual spirit.

I believe that much of the recent success of the theory of the unconscious, or the subliminal, in the religious sphere is due not to its clarity but rather to the satisfying explanation which it offers of the convert's sense of detachment, or of his certainty that he is dominated by, and even subjected to, a force external to himself. The doctrine of the unconscious was suggested by the descriptions of the mystics themselves ; and the psychologists who cannot accept transcendence as such, adhere to it with enthusiasm as a less compromising explanation than that of ' grace '. Numbers of Catholics, especially the Modernists, do not object to this view, because it is an admission that ' grace ' does not operate upon the rational faculty, but only upon the unconscious.[28]

But although the hypothesis of a systematized unconscious can be invoked for certain pathological phenomena, in moments when the consciousness has become totally invalid, it is not justifiably applied to every case. But on the other hand there is no necessity for such an hypothesis to account for the ideational and emotional strife, the falterings, the impulsive decisions, the remorse accompanying the initial departures, intellectual and affective, from the old life.

After all this, it is easily understood why we assign such slight importance to the supposed crisis in true conversion, even though it may be pathological : trauma, an epileptic attack, an hallucination, a sudden illumination, or the fresh comprehension of a verse of the Bible, or a parable of the Gospels.[29] The crisis of conversion, when it occurs, need, therefore, be nothing but an episode in a slow psychic process with conscious lacunæ ; an episode to which we can assign different explanations, not excluding those of pathology (of which hallucinatory visions, epileptic fits, hysteria, trauma, false intuitions, paramnesia, and so forth are examples), but which have only a secondary or purely accidental value in the general process of conversion. The importance of such critical moments consists, in short, in the reflections to which they give rise in the consciousness while being pondered, and in the consent of the will to their content.

In effect, unprejudiced observation reveals the fact that in the conversional process the individual consciousness plays a much more considerable role than has been assigned to it by the majority of psychologists, of the American school in particular. It is, indeed, a fact which may considerably surprise certain upholders of automatism and the determinists à l'outrance, that the objective observation of actions and the testimony of the converted themselves, incontestibly prove that the process of conversion develops with the aid of volitional acts.

The will, as Willenserlebnis, is as certainly a fact of consciousness as is representation. From the psychological aspect the epigram of Nietzsche in Beyond Good and Evil is perfectly correct: " Determinism is a myth. In life there are only strong wills or weak wills."

The convert experiences the decision, the choice of motives, and realizes in action his pre-imagined conduct by means of what we term a ' determining tendency '. The convert, like every mystic, prepares and selects the means by which he ascends the Mount Carmel, in the conception of St. John of the Cross, in contradistinction to the so-called *gratis datae*. Nothing could be clearer or more certain.

The theories of volition do not here concern us. If we were to postulate any, divergencies might crop up among the various psychologists to the detriment of their empiricism. It would, however, not be out of place to state as a matter of history the fact that the *emotional theory* (according to which the will is regarded as a special defluxion of the affects) and the *theory of association* (by which volition is regarded as produced by the correlation of sensation and representation) are both alike in full decadence at the present time. To-day the most widely accepted theory is the *voluntaristic* (which maintains the irreducibility of the volitional into other simpler processes), whether or no this be placed in relationship with the *energetic theory* (by which the will is regarded as an original phenomenon of the psychic *en*) or with the theory of the *Spirit*.

In conclusion then, we find that the possibility of an instantaneous type of conversion cannot be denied. It is not, however, the common type, and whenever it is observed, it is found to differ from the other type less than many would have us believe. Moreover, in both types of conversion, the intervention of the personality of the subject plays no inconsiderable part ; and further, the convert recognizes his mutation however it has occurred, and adheres to his conversion with strong and successively repeated efforts of will and makes it the visible standard of his new life.   It is clear, therefore, that the difference between the two types ultimately becomes so attentuated as almost to vanish altogether.

CHAPTER IV

THE PROCESS OF CONVERSION

CONVERSION, therefore, as we conceive of it, whether fulminant or progressive, is invariably *a mental process*. And this is in no way surprising. All mental phenomena are processes ; in each there is the process of perception, and, particularly, the mnesic process, which proceeds from the ' perseveration of the stimulus ' to the modified ' reproduction ' of the *engram*.

So, too, religious phenomena are only processes. We find the mystics themselves—for example, St. Theresa and St. John of the Cross—describing what they term the *mystic process*, and, notwithstanding the phases which cannot be expressed in words, dividing it into the four famous stages of : *quiet, union, ecstasy*, and *spiritual espousal*, with intermediate phases besides. What may, however, astonish us is that it is the mystics themselves who have given prominence to the physiological stages ' corresponding ' to the phases of the mystic process. It is they, in fact, who have opened to the biologist the way of psycho-physiological observation in the field of religious psychology.

A psychic or a mental process, whether it be cognitive, affective, or a mixture of both, is very familiar in psychology.[1] The word ' process ' implies a continuous alteration in consciousness, or in the mental situation, or in both simultaneously. This continuity can be either in respect of *time* (temporal continuity, devoid of interval) or in respect of *disposition* (which means that the inclination or interest remains constant). This latter signifies that successive states of consciousness may be phases of development of a single conative tendency. A continuity of interest may occur without continuity in time; or vice versa. I can, for example, take up a problem to-day at the point at which I abandoned it yesterday; and despite the interval of time, the trains of thought I pursued yesterday and those I follow to-day possess a continuity of interest.

Whether or not the psychic processes are independent systems produced through the activity of an original force, or in accordance with a law which must be presumed to be invariable, is clearly an inquiry of a philosophical nature which cannot be discussed here.

So often do the psychic processes show a resemblance to the processes of biology that Stanley Hall, as already stated in an earlier chapter, sought in nature for homologies to conversion and actually found them in certain organic mutations among the animals. In this connection, however, we drew attention to the fact that these analogies were too uncertain and in any case too remote to be of any adequate interest. At the same time the attempt to trace a clearer analogy between the processes of ethico-religious conversion and biological adaptation and defence should not be under-estimated, and more especially the homologies between conversion in our sense and biological renewal and regeneration.

Some authors have attempted to discover in conversion an analogy with the appearance of new organic forms in nature. In this problem it is not the creationist theory (of separate creations) that predominates, but the Darwinian evolutionary theory, and Hugo de Vries's theory of mutation. Since the latter theory implies rapidity, it might appear possible to invoke it as homologous to the fulminant type of conversion; more particularly since 'mutation' in the biological sense is preceded, as Höffding asserts, by 'pre-mutations'.

While this is not denied, one should not take too much account of certain comparisons, in view of the scarcity and uncertainty of our present knowledge on such subjects. The Darwinian theory of gradual evolution found authoritative opponents in the past, and to-day meets with still more opposition. On the other hand, the adversaries of the old theory of the transformation of species and the advocates, like Giorgio Sergi, of the polygenetic origin of vegetable and animal life are unable to tell us how rapid variation is effected. They are unable to do more than criticize a theory—which, one must confess, is often abused without scruple—while they still admit the biological unity of the organs and of the elementary functions by which the conservation of the life of the individual and of the species is maintained. Thus, we can get no light from the views of the polygenists—who, moreover, are only a small minority.

Nor do we find the creationists better informed. They limit themselves to admitting the appearance of the forms of life in their specific morphology, without any antecedent transformation. The creationists would be represented in the argument concerning conversion by the believers in the doctrine of absolute 'grace'. It is clear, however, that these ingenuous creationists, who have not the slightest difficulty in admitting the sudden and unmotivated appearance of the various species, assume an attitude beyond the range of scientific good and evil. They oppose every taxonomic scheme which tends towards the inclusion of the *Hominidæ* within

the zoological system. But that some of these negations
—like those of Bomüller, Wasmann, and others—are due
to theoretical preconceptions is evident in the very
words they use in their refutations. On the contrary,
certain postulates may be legitimately admitted by
every sincere scientific worker. Since no one can
contradict that even man is an animal, a theory based
on this admission serves admirably for orientation
in research. To under-value this theory by taking sides
is simply to imply the abandonment of all research.[2]

For our purposes, however, there is no need to go in
search of analogies, either with the creative act, or with
filiation. We can dispense with evolutionism: the
uncontroverted concept of evolution is sufficient for our
purpose, since evolution implies only development and a
genetic nexus in phenomena. Everything in nature, as
Giordano Bruno has expressed it, is connected " in ascent
and descent ". Fortunately the development of beings is
a commonplace of biology; embryology and comparative
anatomy demonstrate the ontogenesis and phylogenesis
of the plants and animals, the kinship and affinity of
forms. There can be no divergence of opinion, then,
on the concept of development.

We may regard the great organic mutations without
hesitation as progress, arrest, or retrogression of development with reference to a somatic type—which may be
purely hypothetical—and which may be either superior
or inferior to the types evolved. In the same way the
psychic mutations of the individual may be regarded
as stages in *progressive* evolution towards an ideal type,
or *regressive* evolution towards an historic or theoretical
type.

The psyche develops in man ' by ascent ' and finds its
parallel in the development of the organism and of the

brain. The psycho-physiology of infancy is rich in documentation of this ontopsychogenic evolution in relation to the development of the form and structure of the brain, and particularly of the neopallium; while pathology confirms, in the most luminous way, the relation between psychic evolution and cerebral development. Thus it has been found that arrested or retarded development of the brain co-exists with arrested or retarded development of the psyche. In short, we can feel assured that the old ' law of continuity ' finds its application to-day, in spite of sharp variations, in the history of religion and of social and individual thought.[3]

When we state the question thus, we can conclude that conversion—considered in the American sense as belonging to the religious crisis of puberty—is a true mental process, consisting of *a slow individual mutation of progressive value*. But the conversion of adults—taken in our sense—must be considered, according to the case, as a process now of *progressive* evolution, now of *regressive* evolution, and either rapid or slow.

The ' typical experience of conversion '—with which we are particularly concerned in this essay—is undoubtedly progressive, not only in respect of an ethically ideal pattern, but even more so in respect of the individual instinct of pleasure, while other experiences may be regressive. Certain ' returns ' in advanced age certainly indicate an involution; yet these one should not hastily consider as pathological, as some would do. We shall see in Chapter VII the nature of the truly ' morbid ' conversions which are not conversions at all.

It may be observed in passing that the conception

of evolutionary development may be accepted even
by those who support on the subject of conversion the
theory of 'revolutionary mutation'. In sociology
revolutions are merely considered to be the epilogue
of a long mutation of the conscience, as the accomplishment of the repeated aspirations of peoples or of smaller
communities.

In enumerating the external and internal factors
of conversion and of the reactions of the consciousness
of the converts, we have only touched upon the surface
of our theme.   In the convert there is, however, something
more profound, which the psychologist must search for
in the roots of life itself.   True conversion is an integral
overturning of consciousness, which gives way to a fresh
psychic systemization.   Brunetière has fully expounded,
with his usual polemical vivacity, his reasons for believing,
but he is silent as to the more intimate motives of his
conversion.   Another celebrated convert of our own
times, Louis Bertrand, declares that he feels a repugnance
to revealing to the eyes of the profane what St. Augustine
describes as the " nuptial chamber of the soul ".   But
it is into these intimate motives that we must enter
if we wish to make a significant study of the effective,
profound, and lasting mutation of the convert.   In
Louise de la Vallière the first conversional crisis was the
effect of a passing shock.   This the Mother Superior
of the Convent of Chaillot so well realized that she would
not receive her as a novice.   The second crisis was ten
years later.   This was a genuine conversion ;   and
Louise entered, and ended her life in, the Carmelite Convent
of the Rue Saint Jacques.   Why was this the real
conversion ?   It was because, the preceding period of
oscillations and conflicts once overcome, the new

emotional systemization of the *grande amoureuse* was at length complete.

Not in all converts are the affective depths so quickly explored. Moreover, it is certain that each conversion contains a certain element of originality, although the analysis of typical cases may suggest certain generalizations.

It is certain that conversion does not imply in all cases and everywhere the equivalent of a lasting life of moral perfection. In many instances the conversion becomes exhausted by a period of affective and philosophic oscillations, ending in a series of practical compromises. But in all true conversions there is a moment—no matter how fleeting—during which the mutation extends to the profoundest roots of the affective life, though it may have seemed to involve only the intelligence. Every conversion, therefore, is to be considered as a new psychic systemization

This brings us to a critical point in our train of argument, and it is indispensable to halt here in order to clarify certain points.

I. *Psychic Systems or Complexes*

It is here necessary to lay down a scheme of psychological dynamics. We shall have frequent occasion to refer to the ideas of Sigmund Freud, because we are convinced that to-day no one can undertake any work in individual psychology without seriously considering his theories. This does not necessarily involve the application of psycho-analysis in any partisan spirit to the psychology of religion ; nor does it necessitate ignoring the work of Freud's predecessors, Janet or Paulhan, or the researches of his epigones. It means simply that we shall utilize the very important contributions which we owe to that author in this particular branch of modern psychology. In any case, we want to take account especially of the modern development of psychology, and to note all the new currents which are working from different directions to effect a reform in the fundamental conception of the psyche.

It is now impossible not to conceive of the psyche in the dynamic sense, as a play of forces. Everything in us unfolds itself and flows in accordance with the conception of William James, of a *stream of thought*. For the rest, even in the older literature one finds the expressions ' psychic force ', ' psychological tension ', ' the psychic potential ', and so forth. Thus, for example, that a tendency was a potential of action or a tension was implicit in the Aristotelian conception of ὄρεξις (Aristotle, *Rhet.* I, 10, 3) ; but the development of such a conception came with the study of the unconscious (dynamic unconscious). The difference between the point of view of the physiologists, psychologists, and psycho-pathologists who have adopted the nomenclature of physics, and ourselves, is this : that they, like Haeckel, either committed the inexcusable error of confounding energy in general with the soul or with the spirit, and were, therefore, led to recognize a soul or a spirit in all matter ; or else they postulated psychic activity as one of the forms of energy, thus unconsciously preparing a philosophy for psychologists which was more or less Ostwald's theory of ' Energetics ' ; or again, with Höfler, they endeavoured to maintain that the human soul was a closed system, absolutely incapable of giving off or of borrowing new energy from any external system, thus affirming not only a fact (which appears to everyone indisputable), but a metaphysical theory respecting the nature of energy itself.

We, on the contrary, shall adopt the same nomenclature of psychic energy, tension, psychic potential, and so forth, but do not renounce the conception that the human psyche is a form of activity *sui generis*, regarding whose essence and origin the science of psychology remains, and should remain, entirely agnostic. We can only know this in regard to it : that this force works with the energy (which has also its unknown principles) which we call physico-chemical (or perhaps biological or vital or nervous)—though it is not on that account to be confused with this, as is the mental habit of many neurologists. The psyche has been variously explained as a condensation of potential by the cerebral cells with short axons ; or as electric currents of the nervous tissue ; or as the solution and precipitation of colloidal substances . . . and so on. The psychologist may not know, but the philosopher knows for him ! For the philosopher everything is clear, even though what for him is clarity and truth may appear to be obscurity and error for another.

Psychic energy,[4] then, besides its diverse names, assumes ' aspects ' and ' gradations ' of varying importance. It is by reason of psychic energy that I feel and imagine and value myself ; that I can reason and will. I, therefore, actually am energy. Imagination, intelligence, and will are certainly forms of psychic energy, but they are different aspects of it. Moreover, the associated physico-chemical energy enters into and influences to a varying degree the different conditions of the conscious and the subconscious : dominant in the realm of the feelings ; scarcely perceptible, though always present, in the reason.

This implies that the two curves of energy—the psychic and the vital (vital is here used in the purely physiological sense)—sometimes run with a certain parallelism and sometimes do not, and yet that they always maintain the magnificent proportion which constitutes the harmony between life and thought.

It may here be usefully repeated that psychic energy also animates the contents of the subconscious, the instincts, the tendencies, the habits ; and that, therefore, the subconscious possesses its own dynamic forces, which it continually manifests in dreams, in movement, in gestures, in speech, and in humour. So too, what Marbe calls the *Bewusstseinslage*, and what the Americans and the French call *attitude* is only psychic energy, with its associated vital force. In the same way, what Janet [5] terms ' psychological tension ' is purely psychological ; and the potential to which Bianchi so often alludes in his books is—in my opinion—psychic potential connected with its physico-chemical associate and not psychic alone. Every discussion of the nature of ' attitude ' seems to me futile, since this cannot possibly be *nervous only*, or *psychic only*, except at the cost of introducing into the sphere of scientific psychology— and accepting—a distinctively philosophical conception of causality.[6]

As in the world of physics, life, and economics, struggle and competition exist also in the psychic realm. This struggle appears in displacements of energy. In fact psychic energy does not animate at every moment and in the same degree the diverse psychic forms, the affective states, the tendencies, instincts, memories, judgments, and so forth. It is constantly undergoing displacement, like a reflection mirrored on water agitated by the wind. In its manifestation as self-consciousness and will, psychic energy is capable, under certain conditions and up to a certain point, of directing its own displacements. When this auto-direction becomes defective, the result is either an eclipse of the consciousness, or automatism, or semi-automatic habits, or those more or less stable deviations of energy which we term psychic maladies or anomalies. These deviations are not only associated with cerebral concomitants, but are definitely provoked by physico-chemical, histological, or anatomical changes occurring in the nervous system. Be it said in passing, but with due emphasis, a mental disorder without a pathological cerebral provocation is unthinkable for a man of science.

It is easy to imagine that everything that exists in our subconscious mind, as well as everything we consciously think or perform, is charged with psychic activity or energy. It is, moreover, easy to deduce that a ' psychic charge ' exists also in the elementary psychic contents, such as perception and representation. But this energy is concentrated upon the psychic complexes in which representation is associated with the affects and impulses.

Actually we feel, perceive, remember, or think, not by those simple elements which analysis shows us, but by a synthetic process. The material of our perception, memory, and thought consists of minute planetary systems, akin to the atoms of modern chemistry, and not of indivisable elements like the electron. As a consequence of this, even our past experiences, whether personal, family, or hereditary, seethe in our subconscious in the form of dispositions which, blossoming in the consciousness, become complex ' constellations ' or psychic ' syntheses '. It is to be concluded, therefore, that the *psychic unit* is neither the image itself, nor the constellation of several images, nor the synthetic image, nor yet the pure affect, but a representational-affective-

H

motor grouping, to which we give the name of a
' psychic system ', or to employ the terminology of Jung
and Bleuler, now in constant usage, a *complexus* or
' complex '.[7]

This, indeed, is no new conception in contemporary
psychology.[8] Wundt [9] held that all the elements of our
consciousness are combined among themselves. The
beats of a metronome, which are isolated, are combined
by us into a rhythmic unity, by means of our sense
of tension and of relaxation, and of the concomitant
muscular sensations. He is of opinion that all ideational
compounds, complex feelings, emotions, and volitional
processes are the effects of psychic processes of combination. The laws of these combinations are precisely
the same as those of association ; whence it follows that
we think by systems or complexes.

It is not the separate, almost pulverized sensations
and images agitated by the wind of association, which
constitute conscious or subconscious psychic activity.
Our mind is not, as Hippolyte Taine has said, ' a polyp
of images '; nor is it a ' universe of representations ',
as Herbart imagines ; nor a ' mosaic ', or in other words,
a sum of elementary contents, or a co-ordinated summa-
tion (*Unsummenhafte*). In reality, the psychic life is
dominated by the motor activity that forms part of
psychic groups or wholes, which are thus active
or dynamic, not only when they emerge upwards into
the light of consciousness, but are also active, to a varying
degree, even when they lie hidden or obscure as various
kinds of dispositions within the sphere of the subconscious, or as others call it, the unconscious.

In fact, the psychic units within us are not cold and
static representational constellations, but are ' systems '—
tiny psychological organisms, according to Paulhan's

conception, made up of representational, affective, and motor elements.

This conception is justified not only by introspection and experiment, but also by considerations of analogy. The simple atom—which one may consider as the unit of matter and energy—resembles in its structure and movements our solar system. More complex still is the compound atom, which may be compared to several solar systems held together by a hypothetical centre of attraction. The molecule—another physical unit—and the cell unit of biology, are the centres of exceedingly complicated forces. No wonder, then, that the unit of psychology consists of the complex, or psychic system, although analysis can resolve it into more subtle elements.

These psychic systems are continually breaking up. Whether they operate in the subconscious, or whether they form the conscious content, the psychic systems are incessantly subject to dissociative and analytical processes—as we are to see farther on—in exactly the same way as matter is decomposed into ions in electrolysis. If in these processes energy has been liberated, it is also certain that there remains in the dissociated elements energy sufficient to determine ever new compositions and combinations.

This must not be misunderstood by the reader. It is not implied that universal attraction and chemical and colloidal affinity possess the same nature as vital energy, or that vital energy is the same as psychic energy. All such controversial considerations must be ignored by the empirical psychologist. All that is here attempted is to emphasize the conception that everything in nature is energized in form and direction by powerful forces ; and it would be to misunderstand the psyche to attempt to reduce its elements to simple autonomous representations.

In the depths of our conscious or unconscious personality, then, these psychic systems or complexes operate. With this once established, it will be easy to understand certain terms which will frequently recur in this study.

We shall speak of ' psychic systemization ', when we find the formation of one or more psychic systems, more or less linked up by close or distant associations. We shall allude to ' unification '—more or less complete— of the psychic personality, in the sense of the harmonious disposition of the subconscious psychic systems in relation to the systems of conscious actuality or the ego. We shall speak of ' conflict ' in the sense of the struggle between the psychic systems and conscious reality; of ' splitting ' in regard to the formation of a more or less complete ' secondary personality ', the autonomy of certain psychic systems which impose themselves on the consciousness. The ' dissociations ' which we shall have to consider further on, will refer to the decomposition of the psychic systems into their elementary components, with the resultant liberation of psychic energy.

This prologue represents the minimum of working hypotheses and of legitimate analogies which ought to be conceded to modern psychology.

The psychic systems reveal themselves to the psychologist at the outset as homogeneous and indivisible formations; or they are detected during the process of their formation. The age best adapted to their solidification in the subconscious is during early infancy—under the lash of the instincts and the primitive tendencies.   But they continue to be formed in childhood, adolescence, and youth, by the action of incessant experiences, which after infancy are more or less controlled or reinforced by the will.   At maturity their production is slackened, as the propulsive energy grows weaker.   In advanced years, we are fed by the psychic capital accumulated during the periods of growth and maturity.   Thus as life goes on, we become less and less original, more and more stereotyped ; we homogenize ourselves progressively, so that at the close of our lives we end by being a faded likeness of our earlier selves.

The modern psycho-physiologist can reconstruct without too much conjecture the biological aspect of this psychic life-history of the individual.   The growth and integration of the various parts of the brain, and especially of the long and short cerebral association paths, support his postulate of the mechanical formation of the 'systems', whose elements are accumulated through sensory experiences, and are fixed in engrams, in close proximity to the sensory-motor areas of the cerebral cortex, or within these areas.   The conception of energy and of nervous tension becomes necessary in order to visualize the activity of the cortical cells and of the short and long association-tracts of the brain and of the nerve connections generally.   Wherever the demonstration of an anatomical-histological substratum is not conceded, the psycho-physiologist can invoke organic metabolism to account for the physico-chemical, that is, dynamic, action which invariably accompanies mutations of histological structure.

To-day our knowledge of the nervous functions is enriched by research into the endocrine-sympathetic apparatus.   According to the subject's age, the single or correlated actions of the glands of internal secretion produce the profoundest changes in the affectivity of the individual, modifying the instincts and tendencies. In other words the intensity and the direction of energy change in such a way that the action and general behaviour of the individual are modified, often in decided manner.[10]   The conscious psychic personality may remain aloof, or it may be present at intervals with an attitude of neutrality, so to speak, towards the incessant changes determined from below. Psychic energy, indeed, is always present whenever a psychic action is performed, and it is manifest in all its fullness and importance in volitional action (but even in this case psychic energy is found to be associated with physico-chemical energy).

This, it will be understood, implies that every individual, at a given period of his life, possesses a heritage of ' psychic systems ' which is at the same time the résumé of his life history.   Now it is upon this psychic material, as well as upon the conscious reality offered by sensory perception and elaborated by thought, that the voluntary and automatic activity of the individual is exercised.

If that is true, it is evident that very rarely will we find men of our civilization who do not possess more or less unwittingly—that is, at a higher or lower level of consciousness—systems or complexes which for brevity we will call ' mystic ' or ' religious '. It does not matter whether we have rejected through logical necessity or lazy imitation the faith, the habits, the things seen, heard, or known in early years, or learnt during the years of education.   Nothing is lost ; this is the law of the spiritual world as well as of the physical.

2. *Rebirth and New Adjustments of the Psychic Systems*

The psychological elaboration of conversion differs very considerably in individual cases. Some conversions are simply a ' rebirth of the religious complexes ' which were submerged but not destroyed. In this case the rebirth of the complex concerns not only the content of the belief, but the belief itself—or ' the state of faith ' —because complexes, as we have seen, are not made up of representation alone, but are also affective-motor. One must remember that representations of will and representations of faith lie dormant in the subconscious. We may be convinced that these representations are never entirely divested of their concomitant motor-affects ; it therefore results that the ideational component of the complex remains intimately united to the feeling-tone, and this latter carries with it the representation of belief and of will, unconscious as memory to the subject.

This is a conception of much importance, not only in the psychological interpretation of conversion, but in the analysis of the entire human personality.

The psychologists, however, have not established this fact with the necessary distinctness. Dreams offer a constant and rich demonstration of this fact, but I do not here wish to repeat what I have recently written on this subject.[11] Instead I would add that mental pathology has been at times successful in demonstrating the existence of unconscious memories of will and of faith.

I may, perhaps, be permitted to refer here to a recent case, the noteworthy evidence of which, it seems to me, is undeniable. It concerns an old lady who was suffering from obsessions, phobias, and anxiety neuroses (psychasthenia with cyclothymia). Two anxiety constellations

filled her mind. One was of sexual origin ; she was
obsessed with a dread of being pregnant, in spite of her
age, and in spite of having undergone total hysterectomy.
The other obsession was the fear of infection ; of infecting
others and of being herself infected, a contamination
obsession.   The origin of these two morbid ideas became
clear to the patient herself at the very first interrogatory
analysis. The contamination fixation dated back to the
time of her convalescence after the operation in 1910.
The other dated from the patient's twenty-fifth year,
when she chanced to overhear her lover remark to a
third person that " science had discovered that a woman
could make herself pregnant by merely thinking with
great concentration upon the sexual act." I wished
to fathom the genesis of this second powerful obsession.
At the second interrogation the following came to light.
It had often happened that my patient had played at
obscene games with children of both sexes. One day,
when she was about ten, a little boy of eight said to her :
" I want to make you a baby."   The words, naturally,
were unaccompanied by any act.   The little girl remained
indifferent and raised no protest.   At the third analysis
it transpired on interrogation that the old lady had, when
a child, practised onanism, and although she had known
of the male sexual organ, she had had no knowledge that
in order to have a child it was necessary to perform
a special sexual manœuvre. The result had been that at
the time she was convinced that she could have one by
simply thinking and wishing—an idea that is believed
by many peasant children and even taught them for
disciplinary purposes.

Here it emerged quite clearly that this lady, at the
age of twenty-five, and on account of certain words
overheard and probably misunderstood. had resurrected

an infantile psychic system, not only with its intellectual content—the possibility of pregnancy by thinking—but also the ' faith ' in such a possibility. The conflict and the anxiety which had tortured this lady for many years were due to the protest of logic against such beliefs, but the protest was ineffectual, so tyrannical is infantile credulity.

The formation of new complexes is not excluded in the process of slow conversion ; the possibility of new formations at any age cannot be excluded. More frequently, however, the adult subject utilizes old complexes rather than forms fresh ones.

It may happen that in the course of years, or in a shorter space of time, a pathematic storm may submerge in the subconscious, and weaken, those complexes in any way antagonistic to the infantile religious complexes. Then this infantile faith—called up again by exterior factors, attracted by associative affinity, it may be of contrast—emerges to the level of consciousness with all its affective and kinæsthetic mass. The disturbance indicates the participation of consciousness in this resurrection, and implies the breaking of habits, the disorientation of thought, and mutations of the affective attitudes.

Does conversion, then, signify a regression to the state of infancy ? In conversions of this type it undoubtedly does. The Gospel dictum, that whosoever does not become again as a little child cannot enter the Kingdom of Heaven, is very apposite. This, however, in no way lessens the ' value ' of these retrogressions towards child-hood. These converts have had to exert much painful force to break through the incrustation of habits, passions, and even of education, in order that a child-like state of faith and hope might again arise.

There is, however, another form of conversion which consists in a ' substitution of complex '. This particular type is especially interesting on account of the intrinsic play of the various components of the complex. One of two things may happen : either the affective component of the complex remains unchanged and the ideational component alone is substituted, or the substitution involves the whole mass of the complex. Both kinds of substitutions may be met with in any of the psychic crises of our lives. Take, for example, the mystic crisis of adolescence which, according to the American school, constitutes the ' typical conversion '. Here, for the most part, we find a substitution *en bloc* ; the series of powerful psychic systems due to education and the fever of sex give way to religious complexes formed in childhood or more recently. The substitution *en bloc* can only occur because the sexual complexes, in certain individuals, have not yet attained maturity and the strength later to be derived from habit ; or because the volitional processes are strongly stimulated from the outside—through education—and are consequently ready and able to surmount formidable obstacles.

Conversion by a rebirth of the infantile complexes *en bloc*, is perhaps the commonest variety. Hermann Ronge, the hero of Jœrgensen's novel, is one such example.[12] At the moment of abjuration he was in a Catholic church in Monaco, when he " recognized that which he had formerly known as a child and which had again become the expression of his convictions ". Two of my cases, the second and third, had the same experience, as will be explained in the final chapter.

In the so-called crises of the political conscience, on the contrary, the substitutions are concerned only with an exchange of the ideational component of the complexes, which had already to some extent been dissociated, or may originally have been but loosely connected. In such cases there remains unchanged the affective component, that is, the quality, the intensity, and the impulsion of the passion, which now associates itself with a new conviction borrowed from social-political events. In whatever form it may be, nothing is dead in us; everything can revive, although the resurrection cannot always be called a victory of resuscitated elements. In fact, there are apparent deaths and purely imaginary resurrections, even in the field of psychology.

The most characteristic moment of true conversion does not consist in the rebirth or in the substitution of the religious complex, which are both unconscious or at least semi-automatic processes. It consists essentially in the ' acceptance of the complex ' on the part of the convert and in the solution which the now reborn or renewed complex offers to the problem of individual happiness for the present and the future.

It is an indisputable fact that all mankind is drawn by the desire for felicity, joy, or peace ; and this law shows no exception in the field of religious phenomena. Father Berthier, commenting on the life of St. John of the Cross,[13] explicitly states that love seeks its own advantage, and that this instinct is a necessity of the soul, which cannot possibly love anything that is not imagined to be good, just as it is impossible for man not to desire his own happiness. The *Euthanasia* of Schopenhauer, the ' death in beauty ' of Ibsen, the ' beautiful death ' of D'Annunzio, deceive no one, perhaps not even those who created the conception and forged the saving phrase. This explains why every convert confesses that the entrance into the new psychological situation coincides with a sense of serenity and joy. The convert knows and feels that he has become a changed person and has the sensation of an entire renewal.

Certainly the acceptance would seem at times to be determined by the logic of the complex. This is only another way of saying that in certain converts the intellectual component of the newly emergent or renewed complex is to be found on the first level. According to some writers, St. Augustine reached his ultimate conversion by way of Neo-Platonism. And it appears that the reading of Virgil's *Æneid*, which lasted for the two consecutive months preceding the final vigil of conversion, constituted the conscious commencement of the mutation of an English convert, Father Knox, as he himself has related.[14]   I have spoken to an Englishman who knows Father Knox, and he tells me that he is a man of cheerful temperament and attractive disposition who embraced Roman Catholicism for doctrinal reasons.

It seems, however, highly probable that the convert, when he is not making literary capital of his experience, or letting himself be influenced by considerations of apologetic, is usually unable to grasp the intimate facts of his change when he is giving his oral or written testimony. Those who deny having experienced fervour, like Monsignor Hugh Benson, are probably not good witnesses. It is enough to read, for example, Georges Dumesnil's account of his conversion, in order to become convinced that it was not so purely intellectual as he claims in his testimony.[15]   The affective component in Giovanni Papini's conversion stands out clearly, though he is an intellectual of the first order.[16]

It must be agreed, on the other hand, that in general the conversions of Protestants to the Catholic Church conform less than the others to our formula of the

' typical ' conversion. It frequently happens that great personalities have gone over to Romanism with quite unchanged moral consciences and an enviable integrity of faith and conduct. Still, I am not convinced that these conversions should be considered as purely ' changes of theological or historical convictions ', as many would call them.

. We may take the celebrated case of Cardinal Newman.[17] Here was a personality of great intellect and of ardent sensibilities ; a theologian, a stylist, a poet, and a man of the most unblemished moral character. In his *Apologia* he relates how since childhood he had taken a resolution to renounce human love and to lead a single life. All the ardour of his adolescence and his youth was directed into the channel of the study and practice of religion. Later another channel for his exuberant energy was found in his friendship for his colleague Edward Bouverie Pusey and his wife, Maria Catherine Barker, and their children, for whom he felt the deepest affection. During the last months of Mrs. Pusey's fatal illness Newman used to go and visit her daily and consoled her with the tenderest friendship. He was present when she died.

As is well known, Pusey was Newman's active and intelligent co-worker in the Oxford Movement ; but by slow degrees the two friends became intellectually estranged because, while Pusey remained faithful to the Anglican Church, Newman went gradually further and further away from it. It has been stated that this estrangement was due exclusively to matters of dogma. An analysis of the personality and of the confessions of Newman, however, will discover more intimate reasons. Newman felt the necessity of a Church which would teach and guide him, and give him a living rule of faith. He

thirsted to have certainties imposed; he required
direction and light. Whence his attachment to the
Bishop of Oxford. When the Bishop, together with other
Anglican bishops, condemned the *Tracts for the Times*,
Newman became dejected and despondent. From 1839
to 1845 Newman led a life of exceptional suffering; he
was alienated from his friends, was looked on with
suspicion by the ecclesiastical authorities, and found
himself morally abandoned by all. We may read the
sermon which Newman preached on 25th September,
1843, in his own church of St. Mary's, Oxford. It was an
emotional discourse; in it he bitterly reproved 'his
mother', the Anglican Church, for not protecting her sons.
It was the soliloquy of a soul overflowing with devotion
which was seeking for an object on which to bestow its
affection, which he found wanting in his own church.
His words to Cardinal Manning: "I love the Church of
Rome too well", reveal, more than his arguments, the
whole soul of Newman.

After this who could deny that the conversion of
Newman was a love story?

Sometimes negative cases are found to possess demon-
strative force in no way inferior to positive ones.
Newman's close friend Pusey [18] did not become a convert
to Roman Catholicism. He was a profound theologian
with the faith of a child, with a holiness like that of the
most heroic of the saints; he was the founder of an
Anglican religious order, and he remained faithful to his
church while his intimate friend abandoned it. It might
seem that Pusey was restrained from following Newman
by purely intellectual motives, but I am not in agreement with the opinion of Brémond, according to whom
Pusey's conversion *manqué* was due to a hidden ' feeble-
ness of spirit ' within him. Even if a plausible explanation

of Pusey's resistance is to be found in the fact that he
was the leader of many disciples and that he could not
have gone over to Romanism without provoking an
enormous scandal, it is permissible to search for the
deeper motives which fortified his reluctance. It seems
to me likely enough after reading his letters, that Pusey's
love for the Anglican Church was actually the restraining
force.

Pusey experienced love during adolescence at eighteen
years of age ; at twenty he was already suffering the
pains of love, and his only consolation was found in the
uninterrupted study of Oriental languages in England
and in Germany. The woman of his dreams, Maria
Catherine Barker, became his wife after nine years of
waiting, and remained the object of all his devotion for
the eleven years which preceded her death in May, 1839.
The love of his wife and children—of whom he lost two
in early infancy—never was substituted in the flesh, as
Pusey plainly shows in his letters. We have every reason,
therefore, to suppose that all the ardent soul within him
turned back to the old object of his love—the Anglican
Church—whose divine origin he never doubted, just as
one never doubts the wife or the friend one warmly
loves and by whom one is loved in return. What
affective necessity could change and bring about the
conversion of Edward Pusey, whose soul was already
centred upon the Anglican religion, upon which he
lavished all the love he had had for his dead wife ?

At the same time it cannot be doubted that there are
conversions which appear to be more intellectual than
affective ; where, for instance, the subject has never
had any religious education, or where there has been a
Protestant up-bringing.

In this connection we have to reflect that the sub-conscious mind of no individual—even of one brought up in an environment of family or cultural scepticism—is free from beliefs (or 'affects' as Ribot calls them), analogous to religious faith, such as myths, fables, and imaginary happenings taken for realities in the early stages of conscious life. Unconscious hereditary pre-dispositions undoubtedly exist among even those who may be considered as critics, rationalists, or agnostics, pre-dispositions which, under the influence of appropriate stimuli, may arise and assume the form of beliefs. It is true that such hereditary tendencies have more difficulty in becoming effective than the subconscious contents that are of individual origin, as is clearly demonstrable by an analysis of the contents of dreams or hypnotic states, but this may occur, as I have found from the study of atavistic dreams, among psychasthenic and delirious patients. In these the content of the anxiety-neurosis or delirium was not derived from the experiences of the patient's infancy, but consisted of allegories or rationalizations of hereditary dispositions.

One may, however, admit the possibility of an 'intellectual' type of conversion—or the construction of an intellectual edifice of religion—such as is generally admitted. But one may also assert, without fear of contradiction, that the converts in such cases will not be really converts, unless by exercise of the will they con-solidate theory by faith, and faith by action.

The state of conviction is not a purely intellectual condition, as the intellectualists would have us believe. Psychology recognizes its numerous and powerful affective elements, which Jastrow and Rignano have pointed out.[19] *Wissen*, or knowledge, is very often coloured by *Glaube*, or belief. Paradoxical, but full of sense, is the French writer who says that we ' know ' we must die, but we don't ' believe ' it. It might be objected that the convert in such instances trusts in the cognitive factor of his intuitions. But psychology cannot admit, with Pascal, that the ' heart ' is the organ of universal knowledge, comparable in some way to the senses and the intellect, although it recognizes the persuasive force which it exercises on those who listen to its voice. We are also far removed from the modern school of Ritschl, who claims that we have a moral vision and a spiritual perception of supersensible and eternal reality.

We have, instead, to consider in the light of experience and common observation, by what process a cognitive state becomes a state of faith. In actual fact the problem is to recognize the way in which a theoretical conviction —or at least the so-called motives of belief in the truth of religion—becomes a faith sufficiently firm to determine the conversion.

If I am not mistaken, this can be explained by admitting that the subject unconsciously borrows the affective state of faith from infantile complexes, in order to animate the edifice of theoretical religious belief, dissociating the borrowed affect from its content of myth, legend, fable, tradition, and so forth. But how can such a psychological miracle be performed in intelligent persons, jealous of rational values ? The explanation is to be sought in the subconscious. Everyone unknowingly admits that beyond the literal significance of the allegorical and the absurd, there is a mysterious intimacy in which he participates. Only in this way can we explain the fact that sceptics and scientists have superstitions—such as a belief in prophecies regarding one's destiny, and awe inspired by dream-portents.

Thus to the new theoretical religious component,

I

more or less laboriously constructed, is added the load of old belief, living but submerged in the sub-conscious. The complex only now attracts the subject; he voluntarily accepts it, anticipating in his desires the radical mutation of his conduct, in order to win peace and happiness.[20]

In such instances some psychologists, following the example of Myers, would declare that God has worked in the subconscious, thanks to dissociation, while the more orthodox would say that by the performance of the intellectual work of constructing a religion, united to the desire to succeed in it, the convert has merited ' grace '. Both these suppositions, given the limits and the methods we have imposed, must be considered as outside the sphere of psychology.

The conclusion to be drawn is that the affective element predominates in the conversional process; that is to say, when the old religious complex has come to the surface and completed its adjustment by a substitution *en bloc* or of one of its two components, the conversion is still not secure or stable without a reinforcement or re-elabora-tion of the affective component. The mystics, in fact, are unanimous in declaring that the Divine touch is the touch of love. If not all the true converts of history have been exceptionally intelligent, they certainly have all been passionate souls.

The fact is not without significance that the typical conversion does not occur in old age, at the time, that is to say, when life declines. The conversion of Jean de La Fontaine,[21] which occurred in January, 1693, when he was already old and afflicted by a mortal disease, as related by the poet's biographers, is not to be recognized as a typical conversion, although he behaved, as one of them states, "*avec une constance admirable et toute chrétienne*" during the two remaining years of his life. (La Fontaine died on 13th April, 1695.) But some of the biographers definitely claim that he was 'made a convert' by the Abbé Poucet (and not by his own conscience), and that in his two last years he had lost his intellectual powers.

The conversions of Auguste Comte and Maximilien Littré, the two champions of French Positivism, even admitting their historical authenticity, have little real significance, because they lacked the lasting control of action. Perhaps from the psychological aspect Comte's wife was justified in doubting the soundness of his last writings, and in refusing to allow them to be published.

These are experiences occurring in exceptional conditions of life and which, therefore, are outside our province. The conversions of those of whom we possess detailed or autobiographical accounts are phenomena particularly of feeling. It is only the conversion of what English psychologists call 'the feeling-mass', voluntarily accepted and consciously developed, which insures the stability and depth of the mutation, for affective transformation involves the living organism, and is expressed in everyday action.

3. *Affective Transference*

In all this process of rearrangement and reconstruction of the religious complex, there occurs a psychic phenomenon of great interest, which merits a brief but especial illustration.

The process of conversion, in the sense in which we have defined it, consists, essentially, in a 'displacement' of affective psychic energy from one object to another. This displacement is accompanied, according to our view, by a corresponding displacement of vital energy.

This fact, however, is not clear unless the possibility of an ' ideo-affective dissociability ' is admitted. The problem concerns the dissociation of the representation from its affective tone, like the dissociation of the colour from the design of a picture. And ' affective tone ' means the whole gamut of the elementary feelings which accompany representations, ideas, and psychic systems ; not only the sensations of pain or pleasure, of agreeableness or disagreeableness, but also of the so-called ' typical feelings '.[22]

That such dissociations exist is a psychic fact of common observation, to which psychology is obliged to make frequent reference. In hypnotic suggestion, for instance, the operator merely induces dissociation between the affective component and the representative component, in order to relieve the subject of his painful obsession ; he dissociates certain ideo-affective aggregates so as to readjust them in a way serviceable to the subject.

Representations are the mobile surfaces of concepts, while stability is given by the feelings. In fact, the affective state may remain, or return to the consciousness, while the representation to which it was linked may sink beneath the surface, that is to say, into the unconscious. Dante alluded to this when he wrote :

> . . . dopo il sogno la passione impressa
> Rimane e l'altro alla mente non riede.
> (*Paradiso*, XXXIII, 59–60.) *

This is a sufficiently frequent occurrence, as I have noted for many years in this connection. But this, in my opinion, does not fully justify Ribot's theory of the ' affective memory ',[23] although it may seem to

---

* " After the dream the feeling impressed remains, and the rest does not return to the mind."

explain the facts upon which Ribot has based his hypothesis.

The persistence of kinæsthetic impressions, after the disappearance of the representations to which they were united, is a certainty. The so-called ' generic feeling ' is directly derived from these retained kinæsthetic impressions. This datum is increasingly employed to-day in relation to the psychology of memory. It is the generic feeling which guides us in mnemonic re-evocation ; and the mass of kinæsthetic impressions forms the plastic substance out of which our psychic personality is moulded.

We may take the following as a commonplace example of ideo-affective dissociation: I have filled my mind with images of a person or an event, which produce a painful impression upon me. Then my fancy passes on to the consideration of a number of indifferent things ; yet I constantly feel pained or sad for no reason. I reflect and seek for the reason, and finally I discover the memory of the occurrence or the person which I had meanwhile entirely forgotten. Note that on discovering the reason I am either more pained than before, or I experience—at least momentarily—a *détente* which diminishes the degree of my distress, almost as if the success of my search has had the effect of putting something back in its place. If my pain has not ceased, it is because the reinvoked image has revived the affective tone, or has created a new state of anxiety, with its associated connections.

Or take this other example : I get up in the morning in a bad temper or with a feeling of melancholy, for no known reason. After searching, I discover that it must be due to the dream I have just had. The *détente* in this case is definite because I at once realize the unreality of the dream representations; in other words, their irrelevance to my waking existence.

While the affect can either remain in or return to consciousness dissociated from its representation, this does not occur in equal degree with the representation, which, upon returning to consciousness, trails behind it some portion of the affect to which it has been connected, so that it returns with its colour, although the colour may be faded. This is to be explained in several ways: the dissociation may have been incomplete; the tone and the organic resonance may have overflowed the limits of the particular representational group; the return to consciousness of the representation may have reinvigorated the affect already dissociated; or it may at once have given place to a new tone, identical with the original.

The two illustrations given do not altogether explain the phenomenon of dissociation. The transference, of course, may also concern the intellectual content. The transference from one image to another is to be frequently observed in dreams and in ordinary life. This side of the phenomenon, however, has no special bearing on our argument and we will, therefore, pass on.

Instead we must consider other eventualities which come nearer to our problem. Several alternatives may ensue: (a) The image may not recur at all, in spite of all our evocative efforts, or it may return, like a mist for a fleeting moment, but without occupying the focus of consciousness with any degree of constancy or effectiveness. This occasions a sort of irritation of the liberated affect, and in consequence a greater accumulation of propulsive force. (b) From this or from other causes, the affect, on the other hand, may persist and increase in tension and impulsion, becoming finally imperative.

In this event, and especially on account of its propulsive force, the affect undergoes modifications, the most important of which is the following. (c) The affect may become associated with new representations, which it immediately animates with emotion. It is evident that the fresh representation so animated is only the surrogate of that which it has supplanted.

This last possibility is what Freud alludes to as a ' Verschiebung' or displacement ; [24] or what has been called by the author and others in Italian a 'spostamento'; what Ribot terms a 'transfert', Marchesini a 'trapasso', and Bleuler a 'transitivism'. All these terms are synonymous in their origin, but, in view of the wide use that is now being made of them, it would be wiser, in future, to determine their restricted meaning.

In order to elucidate still better the conversional process in relation to its phase of displacement it will, I think, be opportune here to expatiate on this particular phenomenon, which we may consider as an example of the law of affective transference ; a law which, as Rignano shows, belongs to biology.[25] Here it will be indicated by the term 'transference'.

Transference is a common enough fact in practical everyday life. There is a telling phrase in this connection in Huysmans's En Route : " Vous avez des lots arriérés de tendresse à placer : pas de femme, pas d'enfants qui les puissent prendre "—in which the psychological conception of the transference of liberated energy is magnificently expressed. In two recent cases I have had occasion to notice how the husband, after having lost a young wife, found consolation in bestowing all his affection upon his mother-in-law, who reminded him of the physical and moral qualities of the dead wife.

But I have further noted—in one of the two cases—how the object of devotion gradually lost ground; a sure indication that the affect was gradually undergoing a fresh transference to some new person. There are individuals who possess inexhaustible reserves of the *passio amorosa*. They can pass, without an instant's interval, from one love to another; and when the first languishes, the next is already impetuously under way. The passions can be transferred successively to a variety of objects, as a torch can be passed through many hands. Such transfers are frequently to be seen in exceptional men, of whom Richard Wagner is an example.

The sentimentalists delude themselves by thinking that the sudden end of passionate affection between two lovers can give place to a reciprocal esteem and friendship. On the contrary, from the subsiding of one passion there can come nothing but the up-welling of a different passion. Thus it is that from love we pass so rapidly to hate. Hence it would appear to be more normal and certainly less dangerous to pass on to a new love, which is purely and simply the transference of the *passio amorosa* to another object.

Love stories offer innumerable examples of passional transference. Hatred and disdain overflow in phrases and gestures and are revealed in the flushed and convulsed features of a pair of lovers at the moment of rupture. Yet one word of love, spoken in time by one of the two, can determine a rapid passage towards the phrase, the gesture, and the expression of ardour and of tenderness. The passage at times is less sudden, but it is no less tumultuous. One remembers Iseult in the scene of the love-philtre.

The transference of the emotions, of the secret aspirations, of the profoundest needs of the soul, is a matter of universal observation from which there emerges an interesting literature of characters in drama and romance. Catharsis, in the Greek sense, as well as in the definition of the psycho-pathologists, Breuer and Freud, implies fundamentally a transference. The performance of Greek tragedy and the games of the circus were an artificial transference devised to facilitate the catharsis of individuals and the populace. Certain works of art have a special cathartic significance for their own authors, of which we have examples in Goethe's *Werther* and in *Les Châtiments* of Victor Hugo. We do not need to consider whether in these instances we are dealing with an efficacious artifice which is morally innocent.

I personally believe, in fact, that through ' the law of the cycle ' the catharsis may become actually noxious, since by reinvoking the memory it feeds the primordial instincts, and establishes new, but not invariably innocuous, habits. Fortunately, however, there may also be cathartic transferences wholly beneficial for both the subject and the object.

These processes of transference appear clearly in the history of religions and cults, and particularly in the succession of one religion to another. Judaic Messianism, in the souls of the Neo-Christians, became an expectation of the Millennium. The prayer was changed, but the souls of the first-century Christians were clearly Messianic.

The Greco-Roman soldiers in pagan times were protected by the Dioscuri ; at a later date there flourished under Christianity the soldier-saints Sebastian, Theodore, and George, but the soldiers' invocations for protection remained the same. Thus it was that the same votives which were carried at first during the Lupercalia in honour of the Faun Lupercus, the sylvan god who protected Romulus and Remus, came to be borne by the good Romans in honour of St. 'Toto' (or Theodore), the Eastern martyr. Thus one can say that the state of soul has been transferred to another object, and thus while the object changes, the soul remains unchanged. So too it happens that the most ancient sanctuaries were formerly the places of pilgrimage and the altars of other forms of religious devotion in pagan days. Christianity, in its wise pedagogy, left the sanctuary and the rite undisturbed, while changing the object of worship.

The mystics describe certain transfers of love from one object to another ; such, for example, as that which St. John of the Cross describes in certain passages of the *Salita del Carmelo* and in the *Notte Oscura*.[26]

Without going too far back, we have in the last few years been the witnesses of certain individual and collective phenomena which were merely processes of displacement. When we think over the passage of not a few politicians of all countries from pacifism to a belief in military intervention, from Communism to Fascism, do we not recognize the same *pathos* displaced from one system of representations and conceptions and attached to another system ? Is it not clear that the new system is merely the substitute for the old ?

In recent times we have witnessed exceedingly instructive transferences that have occurred in the political sphere. The patriotic pilgrimages, the martyrs, the temples and altars dedicated to the Fatherland, the vigils, the orations, the ceremonies, the propitiations, the tributes, the swearings on bended knee (of D'Annunzio), the relics, the sacred tomb, the Holy Dead (Unknown Soldier)—all those things which have set flowing the tears of so many sensitive souls and which have exalted so many lyrical spirits with pure passion—all these are nothing but conceptions and feelings and gestures and words ' transferred ' from the religious subconsciousness of everyone to patriotic consciousness. We do not lack, in our own days, processions such as those which were made in former times for the transportation of relics, like the celebrated procession of 5th May, 1383, in Siena, for transporting the head of St. Catherine. It is only reasonable to conclude that the intense tumultuous emotions, roused in the mothers and widows of soldiers upon viewing the ' sacred tomb ' of the Unknown Soldier, were not on his own account—as I easily confirmed in several individual instances—but were ' transferences ' of their own grief at the loss of a son or a husband ; that is, a momentary substitution of the object of their sorrow, provoked by affective exaltation.

This is what is called subconscious transference, and it is such, generally speaking. But it is not improbable that, in a few leaders, we find that instead of subconscious transference, voluntary imitations or studied programmes are followed in order to tone down or suppress the religious content, and so divert the channels of the *vis sentimentalis* ; or perhaps to inter-penetrate the conception of the State with religiosity ; or to ' nationalize ' Catholicism.

When we speak of ' transitivism '—a term which already exists in mental pathology—we are naturally dealing with the same thing ; except that among the psychopaths this change of objective has an exclusively personal value, and usually is in some way absurd, or at least inacceptable to others ; or else it is accompanied by the phenomena of morbid symptoms and so forth. Alienists describe various examples of transitivism, in

order to define its character. For example, a patient who
is referred to in the work of Martin Reichardt, insisted
that the persons of his own family, or people living near
him, were suffering from his own malady.   Another
patient, mentioned by Bleuler,[27] had the hallucination
of a face by which he was provoked to terror and screams,
but believed that it was the *face* which was terrified and
screamed, and so on. Here the difference between ' transference ' and ' projection ' is apparent. The observations
of Ferenczi on ' introjections ' are also worthy of mention.[28]
According to this author, the neuropath is constantly
searching—unconsciously—for objects upon which to
transfer his sentiments, and particularly those feelings
which come within the circle of his own immediate
interests.   This is to be contrasted with the typical
mechanism of ' projection ' of which we shall have more
to say further on.

The psychopath and neuropath may present phenomena
of common transferences. But they invariably are tinged
with exaggerated affectivity, which is a morbid sign. For
instance : people naturally love a place in which they
have had pleasant experiences, but the hysteric will go
to absurd lengths in order not to leave it. The innocent
bearer of ill news produces a disagreeable feeling, but the
hysterical subject will detest him for it and may even
attempt to wreak revenge on him. The normal man may
transfer his affection for his first love to someone who
reminds him of her, normal lovers indeed will transfer
their love upon even a letter, a lock of hair, a portrait,
or the like ; but the psychasthenic becomes a fetishist and
symbolizes his love in any object whatsoever—even a
disgusting one.

Modern   psychiatry   has   not   yet   fully   defined
' transitivism ' : it is at least certain that transitivism has

been frequently confused with ' projection ' (as in the case of Reichardt), and also with ' identification ', on which we shall have something to say in a subsequent chapter. It is, however, necessary here to clarify the term ' transitivism ', understanding it as ' affective ' in order to isolate it from the many other disturbances of the personality, and also understanding it as ' pathological ' (in connection with hystero-psychasthenia, schizophrenia, or dementia) in order to distinguish it from the common and normal transposition or transference, the *transfert* of Ribot, or unconscious displacement, the *Verschiebung des Affektes* of the Germans.

But let us again turn to conversion. Briefly we find that in some of the cases observed by us the affective psychic energy of the convert is displaced, and unconsciously transferred in another direction, and thus animates another object which has not been rejected by the intelligence. At other times the displacement may consist in qualitative reversal of the affect, such as takes place in the phenomena of contrast, or passing over to the opposite side. Again, in other cases, the displacement of energy evinces itself in the fusion of all the dispersed or mediocre affective impulses into one powerful impulse—such as love that transcends the flesh. In this way one is easily able to understand the meaning of those statements which we read so often in religious books, such as that wrath, ambition, greed, and chivalry are united in charity.

This exposition then shows us clearly that the displacement of the affect implies the indestructibility of the affect, or of the *pathos*. Is this true, especially if the moral problem is considered ? For my part I do not doubt it. Igino Petrone,[29] in his *Ascetica*, writes that in order to develop the character one must war against the promptings of the senses, the appetites, and the passions, and make a desert of the affective field in order to reconstruct it anew. Benedetto Croce [30] declares with more justice that the passions should not be encouraged to develop but should equally not be suppressed. However, this would indicate that suppression is psychologically possible. We deny this, for the passions correspond to the conditions of life. Spinoza has said that only an affect can overthrow an affect. More philosophical and more true is Lombroso's idea that the affects exist in symbiosis. For the affects and the passions are not suppressed, but are only ' transferred ', ' reversed ' (by contrast), or canalized, unsuspected by the subject, or else with his conscious participation.

But the passions, as we shall presently see, may also undergo a moral transformation, through an ethical investiture.

This is *sublimation.*

CHAPTER V

SUBLIMATION

W E have now reached a point where conversion presents itself a sa concentration of affective energy on the object of faith. This conception, however, appears inadequate and it needs to be further analysed.

If conversion, from the point of view of pure psychology, is a displacement or transference of affective energy to an object which represents the 'substitute' of its antecedent, that is, if it is the product of a play of forces, it does not necessarily follow that the whole process is sufficiently explained, inasmuch as the disintegration and fresh adjustment of the psychic systems occur only in a certain direction, and not in the other.

In fact, counter-conversion, or retrogression, in spite of having the same dynamics as conversion, is a process entirely opposed to it; since besides the actual transference, there must also be an ulterior process which, in its turn, has determined the transference. A passage from magic practices of a purely egoistic significance, or from degrading superstitions, to modern religious cults informed by an altruistic system of morals, may be described as a 'progression', in the sense of being a process of perfection. In the same way, if certain pagan. rites are transformed into symbolic Christian ceremonies, such as baptism, the Eucharist, and so on, such a transformation reveals a refinement in line with an ethical ideal. To this new process, which moves in the direction of something better, we give the name of *sublimation.*

1. The Sublimating Transformation

And what is *sublimation* ?   Certain fanatics seriously
believe that the whole of the new psychology originated
with Freud.   Sublimation, on the contrary, is a word of
considerable antiquity and still older is the conception
it crystallizes.   *Sublimare* in Latin and Italian means to
elevate by the action of an internal force.   This is the
sense of Dante's lines :

> *Come la fronda che flette la cima*
> *Nel transito del vento e poi si leva*
> *Per la propria virtù che la sublima*
>
> (*Paradiso*, XXVI, 85–87.)*

in which the sublimation is derived from its ' own virtue '.

Sublimation, of course, has two meanings ;   the one
physical and the other moral.   In chemistry, the term
sublimation means the direct conversion of a body from
the solid state to a vapour without its undergoing
fusion ;   that sublimation has taken place may be proved
by crystallization on gradually cooling the vapour.

The metaphor has a moral significance in current speech,
drawn expressly from the fact that a crystallized body is
purified.   In fact, the residium after vaporization is the
slag, consisting of other bodies—incapable of sublimation—
foreign to the substance.   Thus we find sublimation means
the purification and crystallization of raw material.

An idea or a moral sentiment ennobles a passion that
is in itself egoistical, or a superstition in itself con-
temptible.   The idea of the salvation of one's Fatherland
even ennobles the hatred and cruelty of the combatant
against his enemy.   This means that sublimation raises,

---

* " As the leaf which bends its top in the passing of the wind
and then lifts itself through its proper virtue which draws it
on high."

enlarges, and gives a social, and thus moral, significance to a psychic fact, or an act of any kind.

The individual instincts or tendencies are susceptible of sublimation. This conception is clear in Plato, when he declares that the love of the good, the true, and the beautiful is only the love of the senses transfigured and given back again transcendent. From the ancient Greeks to the most modern anthropologists and psychologists, there has always been a consensus of opinion upon this point.

The *dolce stil novo* of Dante furnishes an example of the sublimation of love. One may think that Dante sublimated his carnal love for Gemma Donati and for others by means of his divine love for Beatrice, as he confesses in the *Comedia* :

> *Con la predetta conoscenza viva*
> *Tratto m'hanno del mar dell' amor torto*
> *E del diritto m'han posto alla riva.*
>
> (*Paradiso*, XXVI, 61–63.)*

This is a conception that has been re-echoed throughout many centuries, and not only by the mystics and the pure theists. Paul Bourget, in his *Physiologie de l'amour moderne* uses a profound phrase : "la chair une fois domptée ajoute à notre âme". Havelock Ellis,[1] the anthropological psychologist, observed that sexual emotion can be transmuted into a new force, susceptible of the strangest and most varied uses. Ivan Bloch in an interesting chapter of his work fully confirms the idealistic transformation of the love of the senses.[2]

Sublimation, indeed, is a normal and a common psychic process. During the everyday life of the individual

---

* "The aforesaid lively knowledge (has) drawn me from the sea of the wrong love and has set me on the shore of the right."

temporary sublimations, which are automatic and semi-conscious processes, are constantly matured. Anyone who has experienced long periods of chastity will certainly have observed his affective mutations and among them a sort of purification of thought, as though a door has been opened to things ideal. And though the sceptic may be disposed to smile at such a statement, I am convinced that the self-respect of the subject, which plays so large a part in the success of psycho-therapy, increases during periods of continence. Throughout the period of chastity the individual experiences the sensation of an interior force accompanied by an elevation of the sentiments; a solidarity with those who suffer, and with all in need of help.

In every good and honourable marriage there is, with the passing of the years, a certain spontaneous sublimation. The old instinctive carnal love becomes a love beyond that of the senses; it extends, too, and embraces the children, the family. It becomes a factor of high morality.

Sublimation is possible in marriage, even at the time of youthful ardour. Thus we understand how Clement of Alexandria could liken marriage to virginity. That carnal continence with its resultant sublimation may occur even among the married, is demonstrated by the spirit of the Franciscan Third Order.[3] Similarly a rich man can at the same time be poor; a potentate be humble. These things are hard indeed, but they can become possible to certain exceptional souls.

The sexual instinct of many chaste boys, unmarried men, and widows finds a simple substitute in sport, or in manias for flowers or animals; sometimes it is sublimated in friendship or in love of the arts, of knowledge, of the poor, or of humanity.

Sublimation into friendship was clearly affirmed by

St. Augustine. One can deduce from the *Discorsi* of
Fogazzaro [4] that in Rosmini love was sublimated in
friendship. These are the words of Fogazzaro : " Only
friendship could in any way allay the thirst of this
passionate soul, which was forbidden to unite itself with
another soul in love. Rosmini gave himself up to friendship with touching abandonment. When he could directly
harmonize this sentiment with Divine Love he became
intoxicated by it." The exuberant love of Rosmini's
soul shone in his whole life and in his famous sermon on
charity delivered in the Church of the Calvary at Domo-
dossola. I know of an old Catholic who, according to
his own account, never gives way to the flesh, but can
content himself entirely with a very tender friendship,
which he feels for one of his comrades in faith and work.

It is a fact of current observation that, among those
of artistic temperament, the concupiscence of the senses
becomes sublimated in æsthetic expression. It has been
noticed that in puberty the impulse of artistic creation
rises with the sexual life. Every talented youth is a
poet. Perhaps it is to this that Freud [5] alludes in
his *Vorlesungen*, when he writes that the artist
is at bottom an introvert, and that he probably
has in his psychic make-up an intense capacity for
sublimation and a certain facility for repression (*Verdrän-
gungen*). This observation seems to have suggested the
curious idea that it is justifiable to exalt the senses during
religious ceremonies, thereby promoting the sublimation of the libido. E. R. Paolucci [6] in a recent poem
not only justifies, but explicitly advises, such exaltation.
From the psychological aspect he cannot be said to be
wrong, though the expedient is not devoid of danger.

In its evolution the sublimating process assumes
the most varied forms. It can be begun before any sexual

sensations arise; indeed even before the period of puberty, and before the libido becomes definitely sexual. This will be considered later. There are sublimations, also, during the development of sensual love. Whoever has been seriously in love knows that between carnal lust and love there is a kind of antithesis. Respect for the beloved grows with love for her, the audacities of eroticism become attenuated. The German poet Grillparzer confesses that love and sensuality were, in his case, quite distinct. When he loved Theresa he did not think in terms of poetry. One speaks, it is true, of ' integral ' love, as opposed to the idea of ' transcendental ' love. But it is a fact that the two elements of integration —pure love and eroticism—do not coincide as closely in time, that is, in the ecstasies of the flesh, as is generally believed.

Art recognizes that even in love which appears to be merely sensual, there may be moments of sublimation. Leonzio, in Sienkiewicz's *Without Dogma* exclaims : " You do not know that my love has different threads in its texture, some of them purely ideal, drawn from the most delicate elements of poetry. . . . When passion is suspended, I love purely spiritually, as one loves in one's first youth." To keep more closely to our theme we may recall that the converts Hermann and Elsa, in Jœrgensen's novel, have, along with passion, a wave of poetic chastity during their betrothal and also throughout their union.[7]

Literature offers other examples of the same kind. Let us consider that of St. Elizabeth of Hungary. *Die liebe Heilige Elisabeth,* as her biographers call her, was the daughter of Andrew II of Hungary and of Gertrude of Audechs, a descendant of Charlemagne. She was betrothed in her infancy to Louis, son of one of the most

powerful and famous German princes of the thirteenth
century, Hermann, Landgrave of Thuringia and Hesse.
At fourteen she became his happy wife and at twenty
was widowed by his death in the Crusade.   Though
St. Elizabeth was sensually enamoured of Louis she was,
at the same time, able to sublimate her great love into
mysticism.   These words of her biographer [8] are deeply
significant :   " *Lacerabat duris verberibus carnem puella
innocens et pudica.   Laetam coram hominibus se ostentans.
. . . Ad lectumque mariti reversa hilarem se exibuit et
jucundam.*" (Theod. II, 1).

Some may see in this—erroneously—a case of the
usual erotic mysticism of the abnormal or the defective ;
but, as St. François de Sales said :   " Cette princesse était
pauvre en sa richesse et elle était riche en sa pauvreté." [9]
He meant that her carnal love had been sublimated into
something higher than love—poverty, and this would
be inconsistent with the egoism of erotics.   That this was
so, is demonstrated by the conduct of St. Elizabeth after
the death of Louis.   She rejected another princely offer
of marriage and withdrew to a convent at the age of
twenty-two, dying in poverty at twenty-four, and
resembling in all ways her contemporary, Saint Francis
of Assisi.

There is a sort of spontaneous and natural sublimation
noticeable throughout the whole history of love in human
society.   A dawn of sublimation is to be observed in the
passage from sensual pleasure to love, and from polygamy
to monogamy, which is a sublimation by custom.   Love,
in the history of human evolution, first went through a
purely anthropological phase, and then the metaphysical
and theological phase.   In Neo-Platonism we can trace
the transformation of Eros, the little offspring of the love
of Zeus or the adultery of Aphrodite, into mystic or

metaphysical love; in the Orphic Mysteries he had previously symbolized the fundamental impulse of the universe. The pagan conception of Eros was then transformed, and once again sublimated, in Christianity.[10] It is almost a general rule for legends and myths to become sublimated in art and religion. This implies that they undergo an intellectualizing process, an 'affective transformation', with the gradual refinement of the human spirit.

There certainly exist different grades of sublimation, according to the moral value of the 'substitute'. This need occasion no surprise; in the physical world one sees different grades of refinement of the same substance. It is probable that the most heroic grade is sublimation in poverty. This will shortly be considered.

Whoever denies the derivation of pure, ideal love from the lower instinct of sex, controverts evidence. This derivation may be said to be universally admitted by ethnologists, psychologists, physicians, and artists. It stands in need of no further comment. The phenomenon of sublimation, as it occurs in the history of the human race, and in the lives of so many individuals, can be accounted for by the preponderance gradually assumed by the brain over the organs of the vegetative system, and by the continuous evolution of the psycho-social personality.

Sentiment can dominate instinct by the co-operation of the higher senses, in fact æsthetic contemplation and the cult of the beautiful owe much to the sense of sight. Through sight there is formed a mental picture, which, though it may not be the whole æsthetic vision, is at least an important condition for it. Platonic philosophy, both in Greece of the classical period and in the Renaissance, began with the vision of perfect form, and the joy to be derived from its contemplation. What Nietzsche has to say on this subject is profoundly true: that without the exasperation of the sexual system we could have had no Raphael.

There are, of course, innumerable witnesses in confirmation of the common origin of love—sexual, ideal, and divine—and particularly of the derivation of the last from the first, by means of the process of sublimation. First Origen, then St. Bernard, Richard of St. Victor, and many others are in mystic agreement with the *Song of Songs*. We find divine love described in human terms in the *Imitation of Christ*. There is a brutal eloquence in the phrase of St. Bonaventura regarding St. Francis: "Franciscus castravit se et eunuchizavit propter regnum coelorum."

We read in the *Fioretti di San Francesco* of a friar who would have been driven to leave the Order by the force of his temptations of the flesh, had he not approached Brother Simon. "The ardour of his temptation was transmuted into ardour for the Holy Spirit, because he was kindled by that flaming coal, who was Friar Simon, so that he became inflamed with the love of God and of his neighbour." [11]

In the loftiest mystic states of all religions and of all times we find mention of 'union', of divine espousals, of marriage. St. John of the Cross employs a terminology of impressive psychological precision: "The soul", he declares, "which is enamoured lacks the things of nature, but soon, supernaturally, it is infused with the divine. God never leaves an emptiness without filling it." And the same mystic,[12] commenting on the phrase, 'the Night of Darkness', analogizes the three nights of the soul's waiting before it attains to 'union', with the three nights which the angel commanded Tobias to tarry before union with his spouse. So much appearance of sensuality had the mysticism of St. Theresa that the theologian, Gaspar Daza of Avila, doubted whether it was not the work of the devil. St. Catherine of Siena used expressions that could be called erotic. St. Gertrude said of Jesus: "loving, but purely; touching, but chastely; receiving, but virginally." [13] Indeed, we could not understand why mystics have always assigned the highest place to the virtue of chastity, unless it were admitted that they repressed the flesh with benefit to the spirit. The spiritual proverb attributed to St. John of the Cross is also eloquent testimony: "Gustato spiritu desipit omnis caro."

The decided influence of the renunciation of the flesh on the development of the spirit is expounded in the *Fioretti*.[14] In the chapter on *Sancta Chastitade* Frate Egidio replies to his brother: "The most suave chastity possesses certain perfections in itself; but none other virtue can possess any perfection if it be without chastity." In the sonnet of Brother Egidio we read:

> *O santa castità . . .*
> *Chi non ti assaggia non sa quanto vale.*
> *Però gli stolti non conoscono il tuo valore.*

But besides this, mystic love, in the process of sublimation, carries over carnal love in all its varied moods and intensity. It is not difficult to discover in divine and ideal love the sadistic or masochistic promptings of carnal love: poverty longed for, willed, enjoyed in all its asperities and with all its renunciations; the discipline, the fastings, the martyrdoms, the lacerations, the wounds, the wailings, the anguish of sufferings desired or realized.

This, surely, is expressed in the words of Jacopone da Todi :

Fac me plagis vulnerari,
Fac me cruce inebriari,
Et Cruore filii ?

These are remarkable practices, recalling the aberrations and degenerations of sensuality, and assuming a sense of nobility and greatness only by virtue of their transformation through sublimation.

We must emphasize our contention that ardent love animates the souls of all mystics and great converts, which attests its source deep in the sphere of the instincts. I am not sure that we can support historically the theory that the wholly chaste but tender relationships of St. Clara and St. Francis, of Bl. Giovanni Colombini and Madonna Paola Foresia, of St. Gaetano of Tiene and Laura Mignani, of St. François de Sales and Madame de Chantal, were sublimations, spontaneous or volitional ; but nothing prevents us from regarding them as different from ordinary, simple friendships. Every one of these instances demonstrates the ardour which animated these devout souls. St. Theresa, that great passional soul, confessed that she never felt the least attraction towards anything that might make her lose her innocence. Yet her attachment to Father Graziano was at times accompanied by strong emotions which, if they did not move her senses, moved her heart, as the saint herself confesses. It was an affection not comparable to that between women, but rather to that which exists between a father and daughter.[15] If St. Catherine of Siena [16] can say of herself, ' my nature is fire ', it may be asked how these perennial flames could burn outside of carnal love. The fires of nature are not put out except by

natural causes—that is to say, by illness and senility;
but if these two conditions are absent, we must surmise
that the inextinguishable fire burns on, feeding itself,
not on the flesh, but on ideas.

The Renaissance encouraged these sublimations of
love. Take as a single example the case of St. Gaetano
of Tiene.[17] The Renaissance attempted to adapt
Christianity to life; and although it appeared to fanatics
and zealots a return to paganism, and was for corrupt
souls a period of sheer paganism, to Christian souls it
meant the sublimation of the joy of life. The same thing
had occurred in the thirteenth century. St. Francis
was a herald of love. In Florence, at that time, there
might have been seen companies of hundreds of white-
robed people, going through the streets, preceded by
trumpets and led by a chief, who was called the Lord of
Love. And what were the *Paradiso* and the *Vita Nova*
but outpourings of love?

Thus the fifteenth and sixteenth centuries merely
reaped their heritage. Sadoleto proclaimed clearly in
those times that love is the first and greatest cause of our
salvation. The theme of Cardinal Bembo, in the speech
at the end of the *Cortigiano perfetto* of Castiglione, and
in the *Asolani* is this: that all love is one; that the love
of the individual merges into ideal love; and that ideal
love merges into divine. The same conception occurs in
Bl. Card. Bellarmine;[18] and even in St. François de
Sales, in his *Traité de l'amour de Dieu*. The more modern
form of this belief is to be found in the cult of the Sacred
Heart, which is a crystallization of the popular form
of mystic love.

In Rome, before 1500, there flourished the Society
or Sodality of Divine Love, dominated by Sadoleto and
St. Gaetano of Tiene, with ramifications throughout

the whole of Italy. We can picture the reunions of these enthusiasts, who discoursed on beauty and goodness in the tiny church of San Silvestro e Dorotea in Trastevere, beneath the Janiculum ; founding, in a lyrical sublimation, the Renaissance of Rome with divine love.

St. Gaetano ardently loved Laura Mignani, an Augustinian nun at Brescia, whom he had never seen. It was love, not friendship ; that love which is, above the senses, and is purified of carnal desires. Though this love was sublimated it was none the less intense, as is shown by his letters to her, and most of all by his famous vision of Christmas night, 1517, in the church of St. Maria Maggiore. The content of this vision, indeed, is not original, for there is more than one identical antecedent case in which the Christ Child has been received into the arms of the supplicant.[19] In it, however, the psychologist sees an allegorical realization of Gaetano's unconscious desire for union with the nun, a ' wish-fulfilment '.

Those for whom this evidence does not suffice may recall those words of St. Bernard, quoted by Joly : " L'amour commence par la chair et il finit par l'esprit." He may reflect, too, on the words of the celebrated Père Lacordaire, who says : " Il n'y a pas deux amours. L'amour céleste et l'amour terrestre sont un même sentiment, à part cette différence que l'amour céleste est infini." Reflections of this kind acquire a more than literary meaning in connection with certain daring expressions of devout souls. Jœrgensen, for instance, to express the joy of Ronge, speaks of the *honeymoon* of the conversion.

That perceptive philosopher, John Stuart Mill, believed that moral and sensual pleasures differ from one another *in kind*. Mill knew neither physiology nor the habits of individuals, and Benedetto Croce reproves him, also, for ignoring the practical doctrines of Fichte and Hegel, who sought to reconcile passion with ethics.[20] Thus the theory of dual origin is opposed by both camps ; by experimental science on the one side, and on the other by pure philosophy.

All that we have expressed so far does not claim to be regarded as new ; with our almost random quotations we have gone back as far as Plato. But the modern psychologists have more sharply defined the process of transformation of the sexual instinct and carnal love. Paulhan speaks of its ' spiritualization ' and its ' idealization '. The first is the co-ordination of tendencies and of ideas, superior to the synthetic unity of organic needs and appetites. Idealization is the purification, or sublimation, of tendencies. Paulhan applies this view to sexual tendencies and also to mysticism.[21]

However, it must be confessed that the study of sublimation is largely due to Freud ; and that with him it becomes a specific process (*Sublimierung*, or *Sublimation* in Pfister's phrase, in place of the literary *Erhebung*). The elements of the sexual instinct, according to Freud, are characterized by their capacity for sublimation ; by their transmutability from a sexual purpose into a remoter end of higher social value. To the deflected energy thus released for human psychic functions, mankind probably owes its highest cultural achievements.[22] Sublimation, as a matter of fact, is a conception which to-day is generally accepted in the Freudian sense : as the accumulation of energy, derived from the instincts or from the inhibited tendencies, in such a way as to reinforce the contrary inhibiting tendency. This is the mechanism of Freud's *Affektverschiebung*, or of the *agglutinierte Kausalität* of Monakoff. Jelliffe, a medical neurologist and Freudian, suggests as an hypothesis of sublimation, that the repression consists in the subordination of certain 'values' of the libido which are at a deep level, in order to utilize the energy so obtained at a higher level in the process of sublimation.[23]

Up to the present we have admitted that the process of sublimation has for its point of departure the libido, properly so-called ; and by that we may have appeared as leaning rather towards Freud—according to whom the libido is the psychic product of the sexual instincts, and of nothing else—rather than to the theories of the other psycho-analysts. We must, however, allude to the opinions of Jung.

According to Jung [24] and his followers, the material of sexual representations can be utilized to create the highest ethical and religious interests. But this does not necessarily imply that the force of the sexual instinct (*sexuelle Triebkräfte*) has been transformed into asexuality. Rather, these complexes are from the first more highly refined (*höheres*), and have an 'anagogic' sense. Thus they are readily interwoven with abstract thoughts, which are rather in the nature of ethics or of religious mysticism, than of the natural sciences. Instead of postulating the existence of a conflict between the ego and the libido, Jung holds that there is a conflict between the task of life (*Lebensaufgabe*) and psychic inertia (*psychische Trägheit*).

I do not intend here to discuss the opinions of the psycho-analysts. I confine myself, therefore, to the observation that Jung with his arguments combats the specific significance of the libido by tracing its deeper current; and that his exploration is sound can be seriously upheld.

Love—in the widest sense—does actually precede sexual maturity. This is observable in the psychology of the infantile mind. It may also be seen in the psychological make-up of those who, owing to defect or absence of the sexual glands, do not indulge in the normal practice of sexuality. In St. Augustine's fine phrase : " *Nondum amabam et amare amabam.*"

Genitality is nothing more than localization of the vital energy of the individual. Sex is an important stage in love. It is, however, a stage at which the greater part of humanity stops short. The sexual instinct, indeed, is only one of the most powerful localizations of the general vital energy.

But in order to make our analysis more specific, let us now go on from this stage of the *libido sexualis*, refraining from probing deeper towards the great mother of all the instincts, the *Hormè*, as Monakoff calls it.

We must consider whether experience warrants taking into account only the *libido sexualis*, using that alone as the starting-point. There are undoubtedly many arguments for Freud's point of view. Not only pathology (hysterico-psychasthenia) furnishes demonstrations of his theory with extraordinary frequency, but everyday existence and religious life provide evidence not to be lightly dismissed.

Love in its completely sublimated form is the all-in-all for saints and mystics, just as love in its more or less sublimated forms is everything for certain temperaments overflowing with lyricism. While Joly declares, " *l'on n'a jamais été saint que par l'amour*", we have also Werther's poignant cry, " Nothing in the world is necessary but love." And Leonzio echoes the thought

with : " Immersed in daily routine men forget, or refuse
to remember, that their sole object is to love. In that
ocean of folly, doubt, malevolence, and uncertainty which
we call life there is only one thing certain, strong as
death, and that thing is love, and beyond it there is
nothing else, nothing."

Since true conversion profoundly agitates the depths
of the individual's affective system, and gives new
meanings and new values to the elements it agitates,
and since the most important of the elements to feel
these vibrations is sensuality, it seems self-evident that
the process of conversion consists in a practical revision
of love. In other words, conversion implies a new
economy of love. But from the theoretical aspect it
is artificial to claim that all the ethical values of a conversion represent sublimations of the original libido.
Rather the process of sublimation must be understood
to include all the old sentimentality or affectivity of
the convert, and not his sensual love alone. The fresh
ethical revaluation therefore has an exceedingly complex
psychogenesis.

Anyone who likes may reduce all the passions of
mankind to their lowest common denominator. Long
before Freud and the Freudian secessionists, love was
recognized as the desire to rule and to possess, a passion
to dominate, as La Rochefoucauld epigrammatically says,
"une passion de régner". However that may be, this is
not the place in which to discuss the Freudian theories of
dementia præcox (*Narzismus*), or the Freudian theories of
paranoia (*Homosexualität*). It is, however, clear that the
points of departure in the fields of both psychology and
of psychopathology can be considered as at least two :
Sensuality and Egoism.

If everything in the convert is changed it must follow

that nothing can be dead within him. For instance, if a convert formerly dominated by the ' will to power ' becomes humble after the conversion, this is not a case of the death of his will-power; it is only a transference of this ' will to power ' from his personal self to the religious idea and to the object of his new faith, which thus becomes ultra-powerful in him. His sense of power remains whole. From what Freud terms the *Ichtrieb*—the ego-instinct—the ' *Ich* ' is withdrawn, and for it is substituted God, the Church, etc. The sublimation here, as always, begins by a transference.[25]

But close observation shows that what remains in the person after the transference is not egoism, but its opposite—humility. The case of the ordinary megalomaniac or paranoiac runs a very different course. Here the process is reversed—the will to power contained in the laws of thought and of life transfers itself upon the personality of the patient. In effect, the will to power embodies itself in the delirious person himself, who therefore becomes strong and overbearing. Adler, in discussing the *Zwangsneurose*, rightly observes that the neuropath will not obey a law external to his own personality, but becomes a law unto himself. This is a long way from the conception of Pascal, who wrote that true conversion consists in humbling oneself before God, in the realization " qu'il y a une opposition invincible entre Dieu et nous et que sans un médiateur il ne peut y avoir commerce ! " Humility, yes, but from a different source.

St. Augustine, Eucken remarks,[26] thirsted for happiness and desired ardently to live : *esse se velle*. Nietzsche repeated the cry in Zarathustra : *vivere velle*. St. Augustine, in fact, superseded Plantonism when he shifted the basis of the spirit from knowledge to will. Human beings are nothing, he said, but will: "*Nihil aliud quod voluntates.*" If what we call love and pride were inherently evil, we should be compelled to regard St. Augustine as still in a state of unconversion after his baptism. This, however, was not the case, because the saint transformed his instincts of will and domination by a complete change of their objective. Had he repressed his pride and his will to the degree of annulment, the suppression of these affective forces would have reduced his actions—as apologist, bishop, and politician—to the level of mediocrity. He tells us, indeed, in his own words: " I am not changed. I have only found myself. I have only changed my path." [27] These words of St. Augustine are of exceptional psychological interest.

The convert, in fact, alters his route ; he does not change his nature. St. Paul, St. Jerome, and many other saints remained men of violent natures. Coming nearer to our own time Huysmans, as Delacroix has declared, carried all his old character over into his religious life. Giovanni Papini — curt, audacious, '*stroncatore*'—who had inveighed even against Jesus Christ, to-day in his *Storia di Cristo* [28] turns towards Him with all the tenderness of which his vast heart is capable, but still reserves his violence for Jews, Socrates, Pilate, and even Joseph of Arimathea. It is exactly as Amiel has said : " Without passions man is but a latent force, a possibility, a block of stone that awaits the blow of the metal to raise the shower of sparks." Nor should it surprise us that Dante, while describing the sublime images of his *Paradiso*, gives way to invective against the Preaching Friars (Canto XXIX). Such things become easily comprehensible when we remember that temperamentally strong partisans have a greater proclivity for conversion than critics or sceptics, because in the latter conviction or belief has to be actually created, while in the partisans it already existed and had simply to be transposed or transferred.

It cannot be denied—and must again be emphasized—that the sublimation of the *libido sexualis* is a process particularly noticeable in some converts. The individual transforms his carnal passions into mystic love, or into the mental, æsthetic, or ethical equivalents of love. His displaced sensuality is sublimated into divine love.

In one of my cases, whom I call No. 4, this is evident. This subject embraced Catholicism not from a sense of compulsion or as an expiation but as a substitute for earthly love. It was a case of voluntary sublimation. These are his own words : " Religion has become an equilibrium for my forces." And again : " There had slept in me a decision to become a Christian for twenty-two years, ever since I failed to realize in marriage that happiness I had dreamed of with my first love. For twenty-two years I had been in a state of disequilibrium ; finally I became an enthusiastic convert and now feel that I have found stability. Carnal affections attract me no longer. Divine love suffices for me and I feel it ardently in communion and throughout the more affecting ceremonies . . . It may seem strange, but it is so : while I am in church, praying with fervour, I feel within me a stronger love for my children, for all things beautiful, and for the person I loved carnally."

In connection with this case it seems opportune to remark that my subject was fully aware of the links between his old sensuality and the sentiments of divine love and tenderness experienced so vividly during communion ; but though conscious of the connection, it did not pain him or depreciate his belief and, for at least a considerable lapse of time, he overcame all desire to return to the flesh.

2. *Voluntary Sublimation*

The psycho-analytic doctrine, as usual, makes the unconscious the essential and predominating element in sublimation. We have already admitted that the process is *frequently* unconscious. But for Freud it is *invariably* unconscious. The *Verurteilung* or *Urteilsverwerfung*—the self-condemnation which the subject passes upon his own sensuality from the vantage of his higher idealism—is conscious, but the passage from sensuality to an ideal love is always unconscious. It is possible that any disagreement with Freud can here be reduced to a question of terms or a mere quibble. It is certain that sublimation may be implicit in the self-censure, and thereby become at once volitional and conscious.

On the other hand it is clear that if sublimation corresponds to a physiological process (and we shall see that it does) this physiological process is unconscious, as are also the psychic modifications accompanying the profounder and subtler initial phases of this same process. But since the conception and the term sublimation are both older than the doctrine of psycho-analysis, the psychologist is under no obligation to adhere to Freud, and this justifies the freedom with which the argument is here treated.

We must, however, proceed by stages. We accept the existence of a psychological process called sublimation. The process is understood to mean uplifting or purification, which we consider as referring to the instincts. We have next to consider the dynamics of this process. It is necessary to establish that a moral element, or value, most undoubtedly enters into the

process of sublimation. We shall see later the psychological implications of this element. For the present
we agree that sublimation—whatever its origin—proceeds
through a gradation of values by means of constant
inhibitions, either automatic or volitional, and incessant
struggle.

Why and how does the person who is sublimating,
whether consciously or unconsciously, proceed along
his scale of values ? Here it is necessary to bear in
mind the rôle of complexes or ' psychic systems '. These
are what constitute the stored up situations or sequences
on which the *activity of the subject* operates in self-
consciousness or will. And we must repeat that if
these systems did not exist the volitional process would
be absent. These uninterrupted sequences constitute
both its immediate and distant determinant. Now the
psychic systems set in motion by the volition are certain
intuitions, powerful even if unperceived, experienced
throughout the generations and in earliest infancy :
intuitions of morality, so-called, because of their social
utility. Such ethical intuitions reveal themselves as
moral to the consciousness, but they invariably correspond
to the ' dispositions ' formed gradually through repetition
in the individual, and perpetuated through the need of
adaptation to the social environment. Anyone lacking
such individual dispositions and such psychic systems
would be unable to sublimate his instincts and passions
excepting through the exercise of the greatest force ;
and should he succeed in achieving a new psychic-moral
construction, he would be a pioneer ; in other words,
a creator of dispositions.

The truth is, however, that these dispositions are the
common patrimony of mankind. It is not a case of
making an appeal to the scale of values imposed by any

one system of ethics, or by the Judaic Christian religion, because even evolutionary morality recognizes a gradation and a progressive development. It recognizes, for instance, the evolutionary steps from impulsive action to self-control ; from the unrestricted freedom of nomadic existence to the necessary adaptations of associated life ; from the gestures of barbarity to the æsthetic symbolism of these same gestures ; from the gratification of the senses to the affections of tenderness and love, and so forth.

It has already been stated that the procreative instinct has undergone a salutary sublimation through monogamy, which is the concentration of sexual tendencies in the desire for a single union ; in other words, through the passage from instinct to love. It is evident that some values are universal and immutable—sincerity, goodness, love of one's neighbour—the moral worth of none of these can ever be denied, not even by a Kant or a Schopenhauer. Only Nietzsche has presumed to trans-valuate all values, and to reduce all morality to the *Wille zur Macht*. But there are very few philosophers like Nietzsche to disrupt the old unconscious stratifica-tions of the human multitudes. It is said, with good reason, that a spontaneous—unimposed—expression of moral conscience exists. The principles of juridics and ethics have derived their finality from custom, and from the habits consonant with social life. Some anthropologists and ethnologists have even admitted, with Wundt, that the primary origin of every custom is religious, since custom itself appears to be informed by the dual sentiments of sympathy and of reverence.

On the other hand, outside of social life biology itself offers a standard by which to recognize the psychological aspect of what are called moral values.

If we see a crude selfishness in animals who provide for their own wants, and those of their offspring, we accept it as consistent with their habit of struggling for their prey; but it is nevertheless true that there are innumerable instances of clear mutualism between animals and even of true symbiosis. Apart from the insects, we see certain pagurians, who allow sponges, actinians, etc., to live and grow on their bodies. Also, the starlings live in symbiosis, indeed in friendship, with larger animals. We have all witnessed the solidarity between the most diverse domesticated animals, as soon as their own fundamental appetites have been satisfied. Furthermore, care for their young and certain social habits, like breeding and feeding in packs, are familiar characteristics in certain animals.

We can trace this still farther back, for we find that though plants struggle against one another for their existence and development, and show admirable reactive modes of defence, it is also true that plants have adapted themselves to animals, and that it is on animal agency that certain plants have to depend for the transportation of the pollen of one flower to the pistil of another.

And if this be so, what wonder is it that certain dispositions of structure and dynamics corresponding to the unconscious tendencies and stored-up situations which we call moral, are discernible in every individual? It might even be thought that in those persons who never manifest them there must be some unusual (gross and somatic) obstacle; as, for instance, in imbeciles, the so-called morally-insane, or the congenitally criminal.

We have seen that the Freudians regard sublimation as invariably a process of the unconscious. But the presence of the ethico-social element as a factor of the process of sublimation, implies, in and of itself, that this cannot always be so. For in each one of us the instinctive life remains strong in spite of the higher stratifications and the stored-up situations, native or acquired, and is not annihilated, or even submerged, by supposed unconscious automatisms. In effect, at a given moment in the evolution of the sublimation, a 'force' is required on the part of the agent, such as the renunciation of the besieging desires for personal gratification : renunciations which are as much socially as religiously imperative.

In this, as in every action, there is something which transcends the prevision of the agent, who, in a sense, acts as if impelled by a purpose not clear to him. Thus it is certain that sublimation has automatic, even unconscious, roots, as has love, and as have all the psychic phenomena comprising the processes of volition. But as love can be maintained, or repulsed, after it has been kindled, so sublimation can be accepted, or rejected, by consciousness after it has been begun in the unconscious. Dante has put this marvellously :

> Onde pognam che di necessitate
> Surga ogni amor che dentro a voi s'accende
> Di ritenerlo è in voi la potestate.

> (*Purgatorio*, XVIII, 70–72.) *

And this is quite natural. This ensemble of obscure processes which are summed up in the volitional *fiat*— and which are referred to in psychology by the old term of 'will'—enters into action only when a psychic process is fully conscious. Consciousness and will are the profound complement of every psychic phenomenon. When the light of consciousness falls upon the act,

* " Wherefore suppose that every love which is kindled within you arise of necessity, the power to arrest it is within you."

many motives emerge, and the perception and evaluation of these motives generate an interior conflict and impel the agent to a decision.

At a given moment of the sublimating process the convert is aware of the great things which are maturing within him, and he struggles and suffers in order that the consummation may be hastened. Sublimation is at once the method of struggle and the solution—now unconscious, now recognized—of the tragic conflicts of the hours of confusion. The overflowing energy is transferred to a serener sphere. In fact, temporary sublimations are of frequent occurrence in periods of social struggle and of disillusionment.

The process of sublimation, then, may be divided into four stages : (*a*) the period of initiation ; (*b*) the period of formation ; (*c*) the period of completion ; (*d*) the period of habituation. The first stage is certainly unconscious and can be likened to the invisible phase of chemical sublimation. The second, even if accompanied by the performance of unconscious work, is, however, distinct, and given value by illumination from the origin of the phenomenon and from anticipation on the part of the subject of its development and its possible consequence. The third period is marked by the voluntary acceptance of the new situation. The fourth period, though conscious, is semi-automatic, since it comes within the laws which govern habit.

Therefore, to dissipate every equivocation, it must first be established that—at least in some individuals, in certain moments, and from the psychological aspect— ' voluntary sublimation ' must be admitted. Dissent may arise in respect of the theory of will, but no psychologist could ever doubt that we are confronted by a *Willenserlebnis*.[29]

The unconscious initiation of sublimation is apparent in the following psychopathic case. In 1920 I was called in to attend a young nun suffering from frequent attacks of convulsions of so severe a character as to be easily taken for epilepsy. From my first visit I was convinced that the patient was suffering from hysteria, as I was easily able to provoke a seizure by supra-pubic pressure. During the fit the patient had a rambling conversation with an imaginary person, using terms of veiled sexuality. I attempted a psycho-therapeutic expedient, and explained the unconscious origin of the convulsion to the Mother Superior, to whom I also said that if means could be found to transfer the unconscious sexual desires into another direction—remote from the complex—the fits would be overcome. At the next convulsive seizure the Mother Superior happened to be present. She remembered my words, and with a fine intuition said to the patient : " Enough ! Here's a kiss for you", and kissed her on the forehead. The fit ceased at once, and no more seizures occurred—at least for several months. The sister, whom I saw later, was quiet and happy. She was cured because her superior loved her.

In this case an *Übertragung*—in the Freudian sense—unconsciously and automatically provoked by the dynamics of psycho-analysis, was accompanied by the sublimation (acceptable to the nun's conscience) of her unconscious sexual desires, a sublimation at least temporary if not definitive. Thus the conflict which provoked the seizures ceased, because the nun loved and was loved by her superior, and because such love is permissible. At least it seems permissible to me, even though we were to admit that in the nun's unconscious the substitute for hetero-eroticism was homosexuality. It should be observed, however, in this connection that if the desire for the Mother Superior's kiss had been homosexual at the time of the seizure, it would have occasioned a repetition of the attacks. But the fits ceased. This, therefore, distinctly demonstrates a displacement of carnal desires—for union with a man—and a transference into a milder form of love, more acceptable to the moral and religious consciousness, and retaining the external symbolism of the kiss. The benefit of such a sublimation is readily seen.

The case strikes me as interesting from the standpoint of therapeutics ; but I have referred to it solely in order to demonstrate that the *Übertragung* during the unconsciousness of the fit was identified with the initiation of an unconscious—though imperfect—sublimation of the patient's sexual desires.

It is not unlikely that *Übertragung* in general actually includes the initial stages of sublimation. It is certain that the *Vaterkomplex* or ' Father-Complex ' in the transference upon the doctor is a true and implicit sublimation, at least at its commencement. This is better seen in cases of the psycho-analysis of homosexual youths.

The unconscious sublimation of the sexual instinct in infancy and adolescence is a fact sufficiently common. It occurs often among the saints ; at least there are recorded instances in the best-documented lives and autobiographies. We have already cited the instance of St. Elizabeth of Hungary. One is usually assured that the saints—male . or female—never experienced impure thoughts, temptations of the flesh, erotic fantasies, and so forth. Ribot, a psychologist who is certainly under no suspicion, says of St. Margaret Mary Alacoque, that she was *purissima* from the beginning of her life, and at six years old found her happiness consisted · only in praying to Jesus, whom she contemplated in fantasy

with great love. In her very infancy she began
what Ribot describes as her ' romance of [divine] love '.
When St. Margaret Mary took the veil, she was
' betrothed ' to Jesus. As she was pronouncing her
vows the Lord appeared to her and said : " Jusqu'ici
je n'etais que ton fiancé, à partir de ce jour, je veux
être ton époux." Thereupon followed visions in which
the Saint reposed on the bosom of her Spouse, and so
forth.[30] More recent biographers of St. Margaret Mary
confirm the facts mentioned by Ribot. Deminuid [31]
says that at the age of three or four she had a horror
of sin and had already made a vow of chastity—a vow
she afterwards renewed several times—though as she
herself declared in her *Mémoire*, in 1685, she did not,
at the time, understand the meaning of either the word
' vow ' or ' chastity '.

Admitting the authenticity of the facts, we must
suppose that in the later childhood of St. Margaret
Mary it was a case of the unconscious sublimation of
the normal eroticism of childhood, or—what appears
the more probable explanation—that she herself was,
like many religious souls—St. Theresa, for instance—
arrested in the development of infantile eroticism and
sexuality.

Certain facts concerning the saints are explained
by their environment and the social conventions of their
families, as is the case with St. Margaret Mary. Doubtless
the atmosphere of the environment may be capable of
' sterilizing ' the eroticism of children and adolescents.
Undeniably, there is a very considerable degree of
plasticity of the sexual instinct in gifted individuals,
as, at the other extreme, there is also among the feeble-
minded. We shall refer to this later.

Now what, indeed, is this plasticity ? Certainly it

consists in nothing else than a facility for ideo-affective dissociation, or transference; a facility for connecting the dissociated affect with representations of social and moral value. This, in other words, implies nothing more or less than the capacity for unconscious sublimation. Nor is this view weakened by the fact that even St. Margaret Mary, purest of women, suffered temptations of the flesh during her adult life, as she herself narrates. "I felt myself", she recounts, "so strongly assailed by abominable temptations of impurity that it seemed as if I were already in hell." [32] This indicates that in the fourth decade of her life the process of sublimation which had formerly worked smoothly in her unconscious was halting. But since at each temptation the Saint pronounced her own condemnation, or *Verurteilung*, the process of sublimation was revived. In a certain sense, the intervention of a vigorous volitional activity renders sublimation 'voluntary', through the voluntary repression of the temptations.

We may deduce that the unconscious phase of sublimation is a more or less lengthy process according to the nature of the individual, but is followed in converts and saints by the conscious period, which in my opinion is that most peculiar to the process of sublimation, since it fixes the sublimation and makes it a normal practice of life.

Sublimation is an incessant process within all of us. It operates by means of a 'conflict' or struggle; and, as we have said, although it frequently begins imperceptibly and germinates automatically, at a given period in some individuals—among whom are the 'true converts'—it becomes voluntary.

Renunciations, temptations, conflicts, and even 'falls

from grace' are incontestible proofs of this, since it is
in such situations that the consciousness can recognize
the antagonism between the opposed sets of desires
and the two conflicting courses of action, and in
repentance can estimate defeat, as in deliberate renunciation it can value the victory.

Renunciation, according to Freud,[33] can—but only in
the case of 'predestined' personalities—produce such
a degree of conflict as may give rise to neuroses. As
a matter of fact, medical practitioners and physiologists
are not agreed on the controversial subject of sexual
abstinence. There are apostles who uphold the theories
and the practice of Tolstoi and of Weininger, and recall
with approval the praise Julius Cæsar gave to the
chaste Germanic youth. And there are contemporary
neurologists like Erb who inexorably condemn abstinence.
The truth is not difficult to grasp, once it is separated
from the pedagogic problem. Abstinence, according
to the individual, may occasion pathological nervous
symptoms, or else be the source of heroism because, at
least in some temperaments, it invigorates the mind.
The hero is often an 'erotocrat', according to Hirt.
It must be understood that for hysterico-psychasthenics,
abstinence without sublimation is extremely harmful,
since sublimation is necessary to resolve their conflicts
and restore the equilibrium of their lives. Such cases
can be found among the mystics.[34]

Renunciation is one of the supreme developments
of voluntary sublimation. Truly, as one writer declares,
repressed desires flower in symbols. Goethe renounced—
it is true at the age of seventy-four !—the love of a very
young girl, and from his renunciation there blossomed
the famous Elegy of Marienbad, which was the last
great lyric of this supreme poet. In Richard Wagner

we have another instance. His *Meistersinger* is the epic of the renunciation of Hans Sachs, who through poignant melancholy reaches freedom in song. In the *Ring* he has declared that the Gold of the Rhine could only be won by one who had renounced love—Siegfried. *Tristran und Isolde* represents—if we are to credit Wagner's biographers—the sublimation of his love for Matilde Wesendonk, which he had so long consciously repressed, and which he himself recognized as the creative inspiration of the opera. So Wagner was enabled to proclaim that impersonal love, which rises upwards like a dart, is not less strong than the love which sinks beneath the submerging tide of the senses, and that " great is the force of him who desires, but much greater is that of him who renounces ". In these cases sublimation became the divinely creative inspiration of heroic undertakings, just as in the lives of the saints.

Early in 1921 I happened to receive the testimony of a voluntary sublimation of love from a woman of about twenty-eight, whom I had known for over a decade. This girl, of lively intelligence and highly cultivated, was a capable artist who had been living for several years with a famous painter, and their relations had always been Dionysaic. When they decided to marry, the girl—for quite three months—renounced all sexual relationship with her lover, and in spite of suffering and conflict, she held to her pact. In this period I met her, and heard from her whom, needless to say, I had never expected to mention sublimation, these words : " Since my renunciation, not only my spirit but even my body has been greatly elevated. At times desire makes me suffer greatly, but marriage and eventual motherhood are well worth a great renunciation. When I am seized

with desire I tell my lover, and he helps me. Then
I take all the force of my flesh and transport it into the
world of ideals. It is then that I have my happiest
artistic intuitions, and feel within me a renewal of energy
for my work . . . When I reflect on it, it seems to me that
the union of two people who love one another is something
sacred . . . and that love goes far beyond gratification ;
for that is simply a moment in love.   In this state of
voluntary renunciation I feel happy."

It is a fact of common knowledge that the process
of sublimation frequently encounters insurmountable
obstacles and therefore fails to arrive at completion.
In adolescent sublimations this is the rule.   There is
struggle, after which there is a profound fall back towards
the instincts.   Starbuck does not mention the durability
of the conversions which occurred in the adolescence of his
students.   D'Annunzio gives a masterly description
of the fall of the virgin Orsola, in *Novelle della Pescara* ;
and even in the literature of conversion one may read
of the fall of converts who were not saints.   It is very
strange that the mystics of all times have themselves
noticed the degradations of love which occur during the
phases of its sublimation into divine love.   St. John of
the Cross [35] spoke of the ' sensuality of the soul ' which
occurs when, at the very time of the spiritual exercises,
impure stirrings of the senses awaken of themselves
and pervade the mind.   This possibility he explains by
three reasons : *first*, the senses and the soul are two united
parts which participate together, each in its own way,
in whatever either one receives (through the purgation
of the " dark night " the soul is liberated from this weakness) ; *second*, the devil ; *third*, the force of habit.

There is, and there should be, an education of the
young directed towards the sublimation of the passions.

In fact, religious morality and asceticism have offered, in every age, the expedients which aid in the process of sublimation, and in the maintenance and re-enforcement —consciously and voluntarily—of the sublimation which has already been completed. We can turn to Thomas à Kempis, St. Bernard, Ruysbroeck, Gerson, St. Ignatius, and others, and even to the Luther of before 1521. The means they advise are mortification of the body, physical suffering, and prayer. Terence had already warned us: "*Sine Cerere et libero (Baccho) friget Venus.*" Solomon wrote: "When I saw that unless God condescended to me I could not contain myself, I went to him and prayed to him." And the Church in its *Missa in tentatione* implores: "*Ure igne S. Spiritus renes nostros et cor nostrum.*"

It is needless to recall the religious literature on temptation, so familiar to everyone. The legends of the rose bushes which sprang up on the spots where the saints vanquished their temptations by throwing themselves into the snow, or among the thorns, related in connection with St. Francis, St. Benedict, and St. Bernard,[36] are proof that it is painful and arduous to reach the stable and definitive sublimation of the animal passions.

Here there arises a question : Is it rational and useful to encourage the sublimation of the sexual instincts and of carnal love? Let us interrogate medical experience. All medical neurologists are well aware that at times a good remedy for nervous diseases and disturbances of the personality is that suggested by Luther, and before him by St. Paul: "*Si ardes nubere.*" Experience, indeed, demonstrates the cure of hysterical nervous disorders and psychoses, and the remarkable improvements in hysterico-psychasthenics, solely through the well-regulated activity of the sexual functions. But there is another alternative, and it is that devout persons of circumspect conduct should order their life of renunciation by a substitution for—and, better still, by a sublimation of—the carnal appetites. In a woman of seventy obsessed by sensual ideas, and tortured by erotic impulses, I have seen every trace of the neurosis disappear for a long time, when she practised prayer or some other devotional exercise before a favourite image of the Redeemer.

Against the contentions of those who would support sexual gratification as a necessity of spiritual hygiene, and who regard carnal abstinence as highly injurious, one must insist that this certainly cannot be admitted for all cases and for every age, as has already been stated. According to my own professional experience, I can testify that it is perfectly possible to arrive at a condition of mental ' sterilization '—even of the psychically abnormal—by educative methods, without recourse to castration, or to partial thyroidectomy.

And there are still more important cases presented to the medical profession. Undeniably sublimation is imposed at those times when lust has either enfeebled or destroyed the normal physiological instruments. Is not sublimation immensely preferable to the ridiculous efforts of a senile libertinism which is so debasing to human dignity ? Not even the most sceptical thinkers could prefer suicide, or even the threat of it, by those unhappy souls who are compelled through maladies (or, perhaps, honourable wounds) to renounce the flesh, to the alternative of an attempted sublimation on their part. Nor, perhaps, could any doctor give better advice than that of sublimation to the true homo-sexual, in

M

whom the moral sentiment—not infrequently—is very high.

Be this as it may, it appears to me that the study of sublimation should be included in the pedagogical curriculum of the present day. Nowadays there is much discussion as to whether intercourse before the age of twenty is injurious or beneficial; and whether or not masturbation is preferable; at what epoch sexual intercourse is desirable; and whether a sexual regimen throughout adolescence favours, or inhibits, the moral and intellectual development; and so forth. The physical sterilization of imbeciles and throw-backs is also discussed. There have also been frequent discussions and polemics on the subject of the new theories of eugenics by hygienists, politicians, and sociologists. Why not, then, institute a serious discussion on educative sublimation?

3. *The Physiology of Sublimation*

There is no doubt that psycho-physiology could appropriately study the sublimatory process, and, in particular, the period of unconscious sublimation, and its conflicts and oscillations. Sublimation is assuredly a spiritual fact, but it is also, as Benedetto Croce said of Art, ' physically interpretable '.

This subject is suggestive, though it may appear somewhat out of place to the general reader. In any event, I might not have felt disposed to consider such prejudices if another and a more serious reason did not stop me from engulfing myself in so interesting a discussion : I mean the scarcity of data.

At least it is certain that more or less conscious suppression, or subconscious repression of the libido, does

not lead to annulment, but only to transformation, of
forces which then react upon the nervous system and
the whole psychic economy of the individual. It is very
true that a certain antagonism exists between the demands
of sex and those of thought. But we do not know to
what degree the repressed libido influences the brain,
the imagination, the creative faculties, and the intellectual
productivity; we know still less in what manner it
energizes, or inhibits, the central nervous system.[37]

At the moment there is much talk of the secretions
of the endocrine glands, and the stimulation of the nervous
system by hormonic secretions is now generally admitted.
My own opinion, however, is that people have too
hastily accepted certain conclusions.

However, if we cannot to-day indicate the chemical
concomitants (or, to speak physiologically, correlates)
of the process of sublimation, it is because our studies
have not progressed far enough; but the not distant
possibility of a translation of the process into physico-
chemical terms appears clear, when the problem is
precisely stated. The problem may be put thus: Is
it possible that the action of the endocrine-sympathetic
system, under certain conditions and in certain
individuals, excites, invigorates, or refines certain
activities of the feeling and emotions? Does it substitute for these other activities which are connected with
certain representations, which reinforce, for example,
the mild pleasure which is connected with the representation of pure love (friendship, motherhood, ideal love, and
so forth)?

All this is not only a possibility but an everyday
occurrence in all of us, even without the intervention of
the will and the moral factor. There can be no doubt
that the play of the endocrine-sympathetic, modified in

its intimate correlations, or partially intensified or attenuated, must definitely influence the feeling or 'affective' life of the individual. To give a single instance : the idealization of carnal love stands in strict relationship to the age of the subject, in adolescence (by the dissociation of the sexual instinct and the predominance of the internal secretions over the external secretions of the genitalia), in mature years, and in case of nervous exhaustion, and in *debilitas sexualis* or *impotentia sexualis*. In such cases the process is organic in origin and is, therefore, altogether unconscious. It must be remembered that the modification, or suppression, of the so-called external secretions of the sexual glands not only does not suppress internal secretion, but may even promote it. The retaining of such secretions modifies the whole of sexual activity; it does not sterilize the individual completely, but instead brings about a different distribution and a different employment of the libido. The internal secretions of the interstitial genital tissue (the interstitial cells of the testicle, discovered by Leydig, and the interstitial cells and corpus luteum of the ovary and the glandulæ of internal secretion in the uterus) govern, respectively in man or in woman, a great part of the bio-chemical balance. Thus, while they fulfil an office in organic protection and defence, they also powerfully modify the psychic economy of the individual.[38] The recent researches of Sir F. W. Mott and of Miguel Prados y Such concerning dementia præcox tend to emphasize the importance of the functioning of the interstitial cells, even in infants and young children.

The influence of the internal secretions upon the nervous system, and thus on the affectivity and personality of the individual is well known—though it is not yet explained by any theory. The determination of the

individual constitution and temperament must, to a
large extent, derive from the particular manner in which
the endocrine-sympathetic apparatus of the individual
functions ; the suprarenal and thyroid glands especially,
profoundly affect the cerebral cortex and clearly influence the development of the psychic and moral
personality.[39]

It is also well known that the internal secretions, like
certain exogenous toxins, exercise an influence on
eroticism or frigidity, on the tendencies towards either
hetero- or homo-sexuality, on the vividness of imagery,
the course of associations, and so forth.

The influence of the hormones upon the psyche is
indirect, of course, since, as a result of their activity, the
brain is either able or unable to liberate the amount of
nervous energy necessary for the psychic energy to
reinforce the behaviour of the individual, in line with
social and moral requirements. In this light we must
interpret the phenomena observed, for instance, by
Timme, respecting the behaviour of certain adolescent
criminals whose pituitary and pineal glandular secretions
were found to be defective.

It may not be out of place here to note that all
manifestations of the sexual instinct should not be
referred to the external or internal secretions of the
genitalia. This instinct can be dissociated, as Kretschmer
has demonstrated, from all determination by the genital
secretions, remaining subject to the influence either of
the hormonic functioning of the other glands, or more
often, of the whole affective temperament and of the
cortical nervous system. These conceptions are in
harmony with the deductions recently made by Carlo
Ceni [40] from his exhaustive researches into the comparative physiology of maternal love. Ceni, in fact,

maintains that the maternal sentiment is an instinct independent of the organs of internal secretion; disconnected from all the phenomena of procreation; and even opposed to the sexual instincts and functions. According to this observer the maternal instinct is centralized in the morphologically highest part of the brain and is directly transmitted by heredity.

However this may be, physiology can undeniably render intelligible many facts to be found in biography, which certain writers—through sloth or ignorance—declare to be false. Precocious sublimations which are infantile and thus unconscious, as in the case of St. Elizabeth and St. Margaret Mary, are now explained by the psychophysiologists as due to a dissociation of sexuality from the genital organs, or due to an early action of the endocrine-sympathetic favourable to genital inhibitions, retarding the development of genital eroticism, which process is aided later by habit and further encouraged by imitation and education.

It may, perhaps, appear to the reader who follows this reasoning that we are trying to apply a rigid and gross determinism to the process of sublimation; more especially since, in another chapter, mention was made of the play of associations, and especially of the automatic dissociability of the constellation (the representative component of the complex) from the *affectus* (the affective or tonal component of that complex). And yet, after all that has been said, we do not intend to imprison sublimation in the bondage of two fatalistic mechanisms, the associative and the endocrine-sympathetic. We again insist upon the conception of voluntary sublimation; upon a process, that is, which overcomes the determinism of the ordinary organic sort, and whose vital concomitant has to be sought for exclusively in the cortex of the brain. Sensuality may be inhibited by the exercise of fully conscious forces, by a long and dramatic contest, after which the quiet of habituation is reached. Then, especially perhaps in cases of more or less victorious struggles, as the sensuality decreases bit by bit and the external secretory functions of the sexual glands almost insensibly lose their keenest vitality, the nervous centres become 'eroticized', as Steinach expresses it. But the eroticism is such that the individual is purified of the needs of the flesh, while on the other hand, he does not become unsexed.

This consideration suffices to condemn, not merely from the moral, but also from the psychological, aspect, those who because of fanaticism or suggestion would physically castrate themselves in the expectation of vanquishing, by this drastic expedient, an intolerable sensuality. In castration, sexuality itself is condemned with the offending organs; and herein lies its mistake and its crime.

As Origen never attained the honours of the altar, so the mutilated Klingsor never triumphed in the conquest of the Holy Grail, which was won by the 'pure fool' Parsifal, who triumphed over the flesh.

With the little that has been said, we cannot claim to have solved this vast problem. We must, on the contrary, recall how much remains obscure as to what we have called voluntary sublimation. The conception of it, however, should remain. One reflects that true sublimation of the libido is not seen among the animals, though in them the curve of sexuality, under the influences of age and illness, follows the same directions as in man. We can conclude from this that sublimation is a specifically human process ; and this implies that it is linked, not to any decadence or degeneration, not to a state of deficiency, but rather is connected with a higher grade of development of the intelligence and of the social sentiments. And on this the justification of our conception of voluntary sublimation is based.

CHAPTER VI

AFTER THE CONVERSION : THE BEHAVIOUR
OF CONVERTS

THE conversional process has its culminating moments,
its crises. All authors, no less than the auto-
biographers, endeavour to seize upon the phenomena of
consciousness which immediately succeed these climaxes.
Literature furnishes a considerable body of information
upon this subject.

The convert experiences characteristic situations of
consciousness ; but these are not lasting. Their
appearances are fitful ; ultimately revealing, however, a
profound mutation of his entire personality. He enters
upon a new reality, for he now has a new interpretation
and conception of reality. He realizes clearly that he is
not an isolated member of the spiritual human family ;
and feels the reality of communion with all—he is
' religious ' in the etymological sense—and participates in
the solution of the mystery of communion with God, to
whom he is united by the ties of filial veneration. This idea
can be traced as early as St. John and St. Augustine, and it
has received constant re-affirmation from all the converts
whose testimonies I have collected. Conversion is the
acquisition of a new sense, as Bossuet has said. The
metaphor of the man born blind who finally gains sight
has been used many times. The analyses of the psychologists have revealed various aspects of this new sense.

Particularly penetrating is the analysis made by William James of the states of consciousness among the recently converted.

To me there appear to be three essentially typical aspects in which the consciousness of the convert is manifest.

First, there is the sensation of liberation and victory, which the convert displays by a powerful and integral joy of the spirit. One observes, however, that there is a difference between the joy of the convert and the joy of the mystic. When the mystic is in a state of ecstasy or union, the physiological elements are much more abundant and intense than in the convert, whose experience is essentially the regaining of equilibrium and peace after the agitation of the storm. It has been likened by Jœrgensen to " coming out of the sea on to the shore ", or, by my Case No. 2, to " a wanderer in the dark who finds his way ". The repercussion of this affective state on the physical condition of the convert is seen in the clearest way. The convert, if he was formerly ill or infirm, now declares himself re-invigorated or even cured. This occurred in the most indubitable manner in my Case No. 4, that of a Jewish lady.

Secondly, the convert has a sense, more or less like the sense of vision or touch, of nearness to God. It may be that he feels that God has descended into active intimacy with him, or it may be that he himself has become actively approximated to Him. This is the ' sense of presence ' which St. Theresa,[1] anticipating James,[2] so splendidly described, and which—as we shall see in another chapter—never reaches the stage of hallucination. This sense of presence now fills the entire psychic void of the convert, who, though previously subject to periods of *ennui*, or of spiritual weariness, now proclaims himself perfectly recovered. Notwithstanding this, however, those around him observe that he appears, at times, distraught, absorbed in his thoughts, and indifferent to his personal affairs. I, indeed, have heard such complaints from the families of two of my cases.

Thirdly, he has a sentiment of love towards God, which is either ardent or tender, mild or vehement, in accordance with his temperament ; so much so, that in his social actions he feels himself surrounded and encouraged by a hidden flame, which is fed and increased by solitude and prayer. This feeling is often kept secret and jealously guarded, in the same fashion as the passion of timid lovers who long for solitude in which to dream of the beloved and who, with the happiest industry, recall everything connected with the beloved object. But in the convert there is an added sense of ' solemnity ' which is wanting in the case of *innamorati* of the flesh, and which at the same time takes away all sense of shame and timidity. But here again another point of variance between the convert and the mystic is to be noted. The converts, to my experience at least, never speak of *voluptuousness*, nor depict divine love with the glowing colours of the great mystics. In the convert the sentiments of dependence and of veneration are much more profoundly marked than in the mystic, and, as we have already seen in respect of spiritual joy, the physiological elements are less intense.

Listen, by way of contrast, to the mystic : " Now amass all the voluptuousness of this world, make of it one delicious pleasure, and precipitate the whole of it upon one man. Yet it will all amount to nothing as compared to the rapture of which I speak (the chaste enjoyment of Divine love) . . . such joy dissolves a man, and makes him no longer master of his ecstasy. Such delight produces a spiritual intoxication. At times the superabundance of enjoyment forces him to sing, at other times to weep . . . These torrents of delight cause the central forces of man to overflow with a plentitude of sensible love, and the vapour of this plentitude penetrates and reaches the physical life itself and pervades his members." Thus Ruysbroeck.[3]

After this outburst, one is prone to disagree with Father Bernard D'Andermatt,[4] the author of a biography of St. Francis, who declares : " After conversion men may experience consolations which have in them something of the sensual, from which the soul, which gives itself to God, should divert itself, little by little. Thus the soul only exchanges one form of enjoyment for another."

If the convert does undergo these experiences, they occur only during his crises of mysticism, and not during the experiences of conversion properly so called. I know of a convert, poor in mystic experiences, who has repeatedly described his state after conversion as " a peace oscillating between the two extreme points of content-ment and disquietude ". Facts show that converts, in general, may fall into temporary hedonism or quietism, but I do not remember the case of any convert whose confessions admit tendencies of so-called energetic eudæmonism.

However this may be, the convert soon finds himself plunged into inner conflicts, and these struggles still recur after the conversion has been definitely ' accepted ' by the subject. Seneca remarks concerning an individual whom he himself had converted, and who had shown him-self idle and melancholy : " Let him be, let him continue in the way of wisdom to secure his own felicity."

The whole literature of conversion confirms this. Even St. Francis, almost immediately after his conversion, *aliquam habuit carnis tentationem.* He fought against these temptations with the weapon of prayer, but on one occasion, in order to overcome them, he had to fling himself naked into the winter's snow. One might say that almost all converts experience the avidity and the melancholy which the mystics have described. Hermann Ronge, at the very moment of abjuration—which was the solemn final phase of his mutation—was assailed by unbelief so strongly that the ceremony left him cold and depressed. The 'inner night' which precedes conversion here accompanied the entire process, and even followed after it, when it had seemed that sadness was vanquished.

The process of conversion, then, from the objective point of view has, like physiological processes, its phases of secondary oscillations; while from the subjective aspect it is found to evolve in the midst of conflicting motives, like every *true* voluntary process. Not even a complete, strong, and repeated determination of the will can prevent the return of the conflict. It is a fact that the echo of these strong and repeated resolutions resounds constantly within the sphere of consciousness, and that the determinations themselves at last become solidified. It is precisely this fact which justifies the use of the term *true* conversion. However this may be, it is certain that, for at least a time, these conflicts are repeatedly renewed, and the convert suffers. It is, however, also certain that a (post-conversional) counter-conversion of the *true* convert never occurs. This, indeed, is his only privilege.

The various authorities are agreed that the convert never ceases to experience certain painful states which seem to contrast with the joy and peace of conquest; he feels doubts, 'thorns of the spirit,' uncertainties, 'aridity.' If every lover is not subjected to jealous suspicions, to agonies, to fits of despair, at least every lover experiences crises of aridity and conflict. Converts who have experienced the presence of God and Divine love, and thus the ' state of grace ' and zeal, also have experiences of what Truc has described as *états mystiques négatifs*, when doubt, lukewarmness, and sloth prevail.[5] St. Thomas Aquinas, St. Ignatius, and St. Theresa have all described this mood of the soul. Huysmans, through the mouth of his hero Durtal, gives a description of it in *En Route*. The oral communications of sincere souls on this subject are frequently very eloquent. According to the confessions of the converts I have analysed, these phases consist of a sadness provoked by casual discussion or reading, which enfeebles the motives of faith, and which, in any case, hampers the decision to action and magnifies the seriousness of obstacles.

Comment is superfluous. Psychology may diagnose these as intellectual moods of doubt ; but for the most part they are conditions of exhaustion and of hypo-bulia ; hypothymic crises in which the consequent weakness of innervation darkens the mental vision and emphasizes the moral solitude of the subject. These are all conditions which we refer, with Janet, to a lowering of the kinæsthetic level, or to a neuro-psychic hypotension, or a deflection of psychic energy—all of which modern psychopathology attempts to explain by the theory of disturbances of the organo-vegetative system.[6] In fact we must regard the dysthymic states as directly connected with the quality of the hormonic excitants secreted by the endocrine glands, and giving rise to a derangement of cœnæsthesia in the patient.[7] Doubt is an inevitable result.

The oscillations, as already stated, accompany the phenomenon of conversion throughout its entire course ; but they occur also after the conversion is accomplished. They yield only to habit ; in other words, they will yield to time, provided, however, that the will is steadfastly fixed upon the great aims contemplated.

In cases where the conversion is definitely established after the close of the period of conflict, we recognize the mutation of the convert's psychic orientation through his behaviour. The new mental and moral economy recently established in him motivates the new adaptations which he makes to his social environment.

In the biographies of ordinary converts, one reads that after the accomplishment of the conversion the subjects lead lives of tranquillity and devotion. Certain phrases have no real psychological significance. The psychologist will rather interrogate the more noteworthy converts. Of these it is often related that they give themselves up to a life of solitude and contemplation ; or to a life of social action ; or, occasionally, to a life combining both of these forms of activity. This would indicate two different aspects of behaviour : one internal, consisting in prayer (which has been defined as " the foundation of contemplation and the torch of hope ") [8] ; the other, which is internal-external, has an external realization, which is charity.

In my cases of conversion the phenomenon of prayer is much more prominent than is the phenomenon of the spirit of humanitarianism and charity. But in one of these converts, Case No. 4, this form of behaviour was also present. However, it is undeniable that among the great converts of history, charity is to be met with almost constantly.

We now ask ourselves whether these new habits of the convert, namely prayer and charity, are opposed to the interpretation we have offered of conversion, or if they confirm it.

In the case just cited of my Convert No. 4, prayer and good works were without doubt clearly connected with the new economy of love. Prayer became a delight for her which almost involved the senses. Almsgiving was a satisfaction so intimate and profound that it was an indication of a deep sympathy with, and almost a tenderness for, the beggars and the sick who were her pensioners. In literature we find even clearer and more exhaustive indications of this.

It is profitable to recall that in love—and this applies to all three grades, carnal, ideal, and divine, distinguished by the mediæval mystics, by Cardinal Bembo, and by St. François de Sales—the sole aspiration is for *union* with the beloved. This desire for union is identical in all lovers, no matter what their category. We need not discuss prayer, since theologians and positivists are agreed that it consists in an approach to God, a small degree of ecstasy, and a small degree of union. But the actual humanitarian spirit, the love of the poor, and, indeed, the 'will to poverty' of many converts as well as saints, has the same roots as love. It is, in fact, a form of love sublimated.

The source of this 'furious' love of poverty is manifested in many sayings of St. Francis of Assisi and the Bl. Giovanni Colombini ; in Giotto's fresco, the " Marriage of St. Francis with Poverty " in the Lower Church of St. Francis at Assisi; and in the Eleventh Canto of Dante's *Paradiso* ;[9] and in all authors who write about poverty. *À propos* of the Giotto painting we may recall that close beside it is another fresco in which Chastity is vainly assaulted in her citadel, and is honoured by the angels. This does not seem devoid of significance ; this second fresco appears to represent a sort of guarantee that while the 'marriage' of Francis with Poverty is certainly most chaste, it is based upon a sublimation of carnal love. This conception is to be traced in the words of St. Paul's First Epistle to the Corinthians, XIII : " And though I bestow all my goods to feed the poor . . . and have not charity [i.e. love], it profiteth me nothing." Ruysbroeck admirably sub-divides the scale of love into seven grades. While the first consists in having the same thoughts, the same will as God, the second grade consists actually in the adoption of voluntary poverty.

The poverty of the mystics is not the condition of the philosophic life, in the Socratic sense ; it is not a desire for impotence ; in the Christian sense it becomes the opposite, an overpowering impulse, a frenzy of a Dionysiac type, a violence of desire akin to love. It is not philosophy, but lyricism. Thus it becomes easy to understand how the term *mistico-povero* came to imply what the poet affirms, one who has attained freedom. Poverty, in fact, is the essence of spiritual liberty—as well as of material liberty—as Jacopone da Todi sings in his Psalm 59*a*, reiterating the thought of Buddha.

Apart from the mystics, it seems true that sympathy towards the poor has always been a characteristic of the normal convert, which may be considered as one of the consequences of the new economy of love. It may, moreover, be regarded as a sign of true conversion.

From the psychological aspect, the sublimations of love, that is, charity and poverty (poverty being the more heroic realization), are merely *identifications*. The term identification—the *Identifizierung* of the German psycho-analysts—has recently come into general use ; the conception it crystallizes, however, is a very old one, as we shall see, and for the most part coincides with that of *pro-*

jection of the physical or psychic personality, or of some portion of it, upon some other person, animal, or thing. Here analysis discovers certain distinctions; projection, properly so-called, is substitution either in part or in whole of one term, but without loss of this term, whereas identification may be either partial or total, but always implies the annulment of one of the two terms. This we shall explain more fully further on.

The word projection, indeed, has been employed by philosophers and psychologists both of modern times and of antiquity in a variety of different senses, from Spinoza and Condillac, to Ardigò and Sergi. In most instances, however, projection is understood by modern psychologists as the referring of the content of the sensation to an objective cause; or else the spatial objectivation of objects of sensory perception; or else, by the physiologists, the process by which the nervous system refers stimuli to the periphery of the body or to the end organs. Frequently, too, in physiological psychology, projection means localization.

But in physiology and in psycho-physiology, projection is also spoken of in yet another sense. After-images in the retina, whether negative or positive, and those, too, which may be obtained by the stimulation of only one eye, are projected into the binocular field of vision. Thus the optical images which are presented to the visual field when the eyes are closed or when one is going to sleep, are nothing but the projections of so-called 'cerebral images', which, in certain individuals and up to a certain point, can be voluntarily induced, as, for instance, in the case of Goethe, reported by the noted physiologist, Johann Müller. The *Notturno* of D'Annunzio is based upon these visual images, which may be the more readily brought about by closing the eyes and which are more luxuriant and vivid in individuals with a vivid fantasy and an ardent soul.

The reader, however, will recognize that the term projection may have still another significance in psychology. In our sense it means the *projection of representations and of emotions* ; projections which are analogous to those of the cerebral images in the visual field. A mental constellation may thus be projected upon some other person or thing. Such projections are either automatic or, at least in part, voluntary.

In dream states automatic projection is a common occurrence, as Wundt observed.[10] Common experience demonstrates that the persons or things dreamt 'of are the reproductions, or projections, of the dreamer's state of mind. In sleep the projection is unconscious, even in reference to the dream-consciousness. It may become conscious after awakening; but it is altogether exceptional for the projection to be recognized during the dream—in other words, for the subject to understand the meaning of the dream during the dream itself. Oneiric projection, therefore, consists in a pure substitution without annulment, since the personality of the dreamer remains integral, even while it is being projected. Projections of this sort, which are entirely normal, occur frequently in daily life.

In art, again, projections are the rule, being quite frequent and commonplace. Benedetto Croce writes : " The artist escapes from his emotional tumult by objectifying it in lyric images." [11]

Giovanni Papini has made daring projections in his novels and tales ; particularly in the *Tragico quotidiano*, and in the *Pilota cieco*. He kills himself in the *Due Immagini in una vasca*. In his *Storia completamente assurda* he makes the character who knows his intimate

personal history commit suicide—thus killing himself
again. He has projected himself, too, in the *Orologio
fermo alle sette* and to a certain degree in *Il suicida
sostituito*.

Projection is sometimes realized as a psychological
process suggested by the need of individual or collective
defence. *À propos* of Ibsen's *Peer Gynt*, Otto Weininger [12]
declared that a projection phenomenon similar to that of
love is occasioned by hatred. The Devil is the human
objective personification, or *Existentialisierung*, of a
thought-form, which has facilitated the struggle of millions
of men against the element of evil which is shut in
everyone's breast. Aided by the projection of 'the Enemy'
outside of his own personality, the individual has been
enabled to separate himself from evil. Such a projection
is naturally unconscious. This phenomenon of projection
for personal defence appears to be fairly common, both in
individual psychology and in psychopathology. It is a
benign species of catharsis, or liberation, or to adopt the
old term employed by Sergi, an *ecto-phylaxis*.

In occultism projection is often invoked to explain
phenomena—ordinary, curious, or claimed to be magic.
Thus we hear of the ' externalization of the sensibility '
of the subject (De Rochas), or of his astral body (Papus).
By a powerful concentration of the will the individual
is supposed to be able to project out of himself a portion
of his astral body. Similar hypotheses, to-day, have been
adopted by serious persons as the explanation of the
formation of supernormal physical members, impressions
on soft clay, of materializations, and of the ideo-plastic
phenomena claimed to occur by the spiritualists.

In mental pathology the phenomena of projection are
widely represented, but they usually exhibit the specific
characteristics of neuropsychoses or of insanity. Among

my notes for March, 1916, I find the following: A psychasthenic female patient was deeply affected by the fact that her son was suffering from a severe purulent otitis media. Being confined to the bed one day with a slight attack of fever, she declared to the bystanders that she saw in front of her an enormous luminous ear. The projection lasted for several moments.

I have the following note of another, but totally different, case of projection in May, 1920: A neuropathic lady, of the highest moral character, would anxiously inquire, whenever she experienced a mental sorrow or physical pain, whether her son was not also experiencing the same; and would not be quieted until she had received insistent reassurances. She would excuse herself by explaining that she saw every need and every desire in herself so vividly reproduced in her son that it filled her with consternation.

Often, indeed, these trifling alterations of the psychic personality develop a serious pathological significance owing to their duration, since by frequent repetition or persistence they eventually tend to become hardened or 'fixed' in the patient, and develop into powerful convictions in spite of their active conflict with logic and experience. One of my psychasthenic patients, who imagined himself to be tubercular, was convinced he projected bacilli everywhere, even to a distance. Another a melancholic, convinced that he had contracted syphilis, was persuaded that his infection was being constantly communicated to others. An hysterical case was so overcome by the terrifying idea of paralysis, that she was one day found to be suffering from a complete paraplegia.

All the so-called central (i.e. cortical) sensations, as well as all the images of the psychopath, can be not only pathologically projected, but still more pathologically

interpreted. Self-induced hallucinations, which are not
always treated critically, as in the case of Goethe, are to
be considered pathological in themselves. Very interesting,
in this connection, are the projections of ' internal
speech ' which constitute a series of phenomena which
E. Morselli has appropriately regrouped under the name of
exophasia. Certain chronically dissociated dements make
bitter complaints that the voices they hear are audible to
others in the same manner. In these cases the subjects
have unconsciously projected the images of their own
auditory hallucinations. There are paranoiacs who suffer
and become much agitated because they believe they
have been robbed of their thoughts by others. This is
the well-recognized phenomenon of *thought-echo*. In such
cases the paranoiac subjects project their representations, concepts, and judgments. At times, also,
there may be projections, desired or not desired, of the
personal will into some other person, as in the case of a
patient I have at present under observation. This patient
deeply commiserates himself and craves forgiveness for
the ' faults of his will '. On the other hand, a paranoiac
who came under my care some years ago, would declare
that he was possessed of magic powers, and was fully
convinced that he had power to project, at his good
pleasure, his own desires and determinations upon his
friends and enemies; a process which tickled his
vanity.

Many of the well-known phenomena of dissociation,
multiplication, or transformation of the psychic personality, could well be re-grouped under the heading of
pathological projection. In certain cases of chronic
delirium, such as progressive paranoia and dementia
paranoides, it is possible to determine the moment in
which the phase of projection is initiated, and that in

which it becomes transformed into the more advanced phase.

In every form of psychic projection, whether pathological or normal, whether belonging to the sphere of consciousness or to the unconscious, whether completely automatic or semi-voluntary, there are two factors : the subject which projects, and the object which receives the projection. It is possible that the recipient may be profoundly modified by the projection, becoming either disfigured or enhanced as the case may be. But the object and the subject both remain integral and independent of each other, as was briefly indicated above.

There are, however, cases in which the projection annuls now the projector, now the recipient. For the sake of clearness we shall call such cases ' identifications '— a useful distinction, at least in medical practice. Frequently it is evident that the identification consists merely in a *lasting* projection, and is interpreted as an identification because of its persistence in the consciousness. Instances may also occur of the partial or total identification of the subject's personality with other persons or things, which may be either real or imaginary ; these may be due either to the passage of the person into the object of the identification, or to the incorporation of that object into the personality. In this manner it becomes possible to classify identifications as active and passive. Thus it seems necessary to establish, without equivocation, that the phenomenon of identification implies *annulment,* and that this annulment, which may be total or partial, transitory or permanent, must apply to one or the other of the two factors.

It need not surprise us to find that there are states of consciousness which make a kind of bridge between

projections and identifications. Goethe furnishes an example of this when, in *Dichtung und Wahrheit*, he describes
his emotional identification with nature : " I sought to
emancipate myself inwardly from all that was extraneous
and unreal, and to allow things to act upon me. . . I
derived therefrom a marvellous and close association
between my ego and all the objects of Nature ; an
intimate and harmonious union, in which the mutations
of space and time, of the days and the seasons, moved me
profoundly." These words, to be strictly accurate, express
the phenomenon of projection by reception of the object ;
but the elaboration, or interpretation, which the poet
made of it, gives it almost the stamp of identification.

Identification is a very common conception. We find it
in philosophy. The absorption of the world in the absolute
ego of Fichte's philosophy ; Schelling's conception of the
permeation of matter by the spirit ; the fusion of man
with a creative Nature, or of Nature with man, the
creator ; the identity of knowledge and the known ;
and so forth, are all aspects of theoretical identification.
Identification, instead of being the direct product of
conscious reflection, may be a transitory act, evoked by
exceptional moments of psychic intensity, when there is
an intense exaltation of the affective system. It is often
to be met with in poetry. Identifications are frequent,
for instance, in D'Annunzio, whose art is profoundly
permeated by religiosity. In his message of March, 1922,
to the Military Council of Fiume, the poet said : " I do
not live, but the cause lives in me." (" *Non io vivo, ma
la causa in me vive.*") This is reminiscent of the famous
words of St. Paul : " *Vivo ego, jam non ego ; vivit in me
Christus.*"

Identification is certainly a phase of the æsthetic
emotion. Carducci, in the *Canto dell' amore*, says :

E la mia lingua per se stessa mossa
Dice a la Terra e al Cielo Amore, Amore.
Son io che il Cielo abbraccio o da l'interno
*Mi riassorbe l'universo in sè ?**

In the æsthetics of Goethe, *style*, in contradistinction to *manner*, is the annihilation of the poet in nature. The poet, in fact, who feels nature, identifies himself with the light and the life of which he sings. But coming down to more ordinary instances, we may observe how the violinist and the pianist become identical with the instruments from which their sounds are drawn. Thus the conductor is identified with the composer of the music ; the actor identifies himself with his part. There are solemn instants in which such artistic identities may be seen, felt, and understood ; there are even instances in which the composite identification would seem to be extended to include the spectator as well, who, in his turn, becomes united in one whole with the artist and with the instrument, or with the conductor and his orchestra, or the actor and his part. On more than one occasion I have had personal experience of such inclusive identifications.

For the rest, if identification is an accompaniment of the heroic states of the emotions, it is not unnatural for it to loom gigantic in the field of art and in that of religious phenomena. It appears, indeed, in modern æsthetics, under the names *empathy*, *endopathy*, and *Einfühlung*.[13] The term *Einfühlung* was introduced by Robert Vischer to indicate the life with which man invests inanimate objects by means of the æsthetic process. It has met with acceptance by those interested in the psychology of æsthetics, and

---

* " And my tongue moving of itself, says to Earth and Heaven, Love, Love. Is it I that embrace Heaven, or does the universe absorb me into its heart ? "

particularly by Theodor Lipps. According to Volkelt, who, with Lipps, presents the most notable exposition of the æsthetic theory of *Einfühlung*, the perception of the beautiful, on ultimate analysis, is seen to consist in recognizing our own states of soul in the things into which we have sunk them and so enjoying in them our own emotions.

Einfühlung, in fact, for many psychologists, and for Wundt also, implies a projection, in that it cannot be relegated specifically to æsthetics, but belongs to all the active forms of the imagination, from the lowest to the highest grades. To us it would appear that *Einfühlung*, in the strict sense, is a true affective identification, however momentary. It is irrational, and at least during its initiation is unconscious. It is movement and life ; this we can affirm from experience alone, without reference either to Bergson or to Croce's æsthetics. By means of *Einfühlung*, in fact, we enter, through the intuitions, into reality, and in lyric moments of penetration we can feel the contact and the glow of the personality of the artist.

No wonder, that identification is the common manifestation of love in all its forms. In the passionate period of *Sturm und Drang*, romantic love is the absorption of the subject's whole being into the beloved. Union is often an assimilation or fusion, and not a mere projection or joining. I remember the case of a highly romantic reader who identified herself with the heroine of a novel, which she was passionately reading, and was provoked by certain passages in the book to self-pollution. This is a good example of the fantastic exaltations of identification.

Identification is found in the religious phenomenology of all times and all peoples. It occurs in the origins of religion, in totemism. The man was inseparably bound to his totem, which was his protector ; he tried to assimilate himself in it completely, and to assimilate the totem in himself. Indeed the Eucharistic Wafer is a totem which is sacrificed and eaten in order to effect identification with its divine virtue. In the mysteries and esoteric cults the rites performed mirrored a sort of identification of the god with the forces of nature, and with the adepts as well. In mystic exaltations the Bacchante, arrayed in the skin of a beast, became identified with Dionysius, and during the homophagy the fusion was complete. The baptisms of blood in the initiations of the cults of Cybele and Attis are clearly identifications. The initiate who received the blood became identified with the dying god, and when, dripping with blood, he emerged from the trench, the act symbolized the resurrection : *in æternum renatus*. Every religion, in fact, contains instances of the process of identification with God, effected in the primitive cults by mystic orgies, and in the more highly evolved religions by means of prayer.[14]

Prayer—not in its contractual and magic form; but in the mystic sense—is in reality a contact and a fusion. It is through the power of prayer that the suppliant attains to momentary identification with the divine power supplicated. It has been observed that in the ancient religions of Egypt, Assyria, Phœnicia, and Greece, as well as in those of to-day, the supplicants in prayer have used gestures identical with those attributed to the deity. This has come to be interpreted, not as an imitation, but as a momentary projection and identification of the worshipper's soul with the soul of God.

All Christianity is permeated by the Gnostic and Pauline conceptions of oneness with Christ. Christ has risen and lives beyond the confines of the grave. We live in Him and with Him in a mystic union, in an exalted atmosphere. The phrase ἐν χριστῷ ο ἐν κυριῷ is to be found not less than one hundred and sixty-four times in the Pauline writings of certain or dubious authenticity. Again and again : " Ye are dead and your life is hid with Christ in God." . . . " Your bodies are the members of Christ." . . . " We are all members of one body and that body is Christ." . . . " Jesus said : I am the Vine ; ye are the branches."

This conception is to be found in all the eastern mystics of the Church of the first centuries, in hymns, in the so-called Song of Solomon, and in the Homilies of St. Macarius. All impassioned religious souls experience moments of identity with Christ. We may recall in passing the ecstatic vision of the Blessed Angela of Foligno in which she saw the Body of Christ hanging upon the Cross, bleeding and " disarticulated in the members and joints ". She exclaimed : " Pity became acute in me at this sight . . not only were my bowels rent with pain, but my bones were wrenched in all my joints . . . and I was as though transformed in the sorrows of the Crucified." [15] The stigmata can be considered from the psychological aspect as the somatic actualization of an identification with Christ powerfully imagined, and, in a spasm of love, ardently desired.

Does all this demonstrate an immanence in the mystic soul, according to the view of Giovanni Gentile ? [16] If one can speak of immanence at all, it is, in my opinion, simply a process of identification, primarily affective, and not cognitive. The *mystische Einstellung* or mystic fusion, does imply the cessation of antagonism between subject and object ; but this reduces itself to a transitory experience interpreted by religious doctrine, but not certainly in the sense of immanence.[17] The doctrine of immanence, however, is very different from that of absolute idealism, as is shown by

Catholic philosophers, and the theologians of any religion.

Identification must not be confused with that happy intuition by which individuals animated by ardent faith are able to comprehend the point at which all good things, the beauties of Nature and of the flesh, coincide in God. In such intuitions everything, even the subject's own self, becomes an appropriate means whereby to infer, intuitively, the greatness and majesty of God. We may then hear or read such words as these : We are in God or God is in us ; The beauty of Nature is the same as the beauty of God ; and so on. It must be apparent to everyone that this is no case of identification but is simply an instance of ' relation ', grasped with the logic of the heart, visualized and expressed as æsthetic experience.

The Franciscan life outside of the ' halls of the Lord ', that is, in the world, would appear to consist in this comprehension of the relationship between God and material things. For the Franciscans, as for example St. Louis of France or St. Elizabeth of Hungary, St. Ferdinand of Castile or St. Rose of Viterbo, " things have no significance through the natural qualities they may possess in themselves alone, but only as manifestations of Eternal Love ", and so forth . . . " Every good thing in Nature acquires worth as being an anticipation and an effusion of supernatural glory." [18]

There are, however, affective-cognitive projections and identifications either with true and proper fusion, or with true and proper annulment of one factor ; permanent projections and identifications which are entirely individual, illogical, and not corresponding to any collective need or to the traditions which have survived through the ages as serving some useful purpose. These, of course, come within the sphere of pathology. In mental pathology, as we have already remarked, there are to be found all the phenomena of normal psychology, but they are enormously exaggerated, or have a twist of meaning altogether personal, illogical, and extra-social; they are lasting as regards the manner in which they appear, and they produce a profound and complete disturbance in the personality of the subject and in his brain.

The lay reader should not forget that insanity is always a stable condition—although only relatively so, because even insanity may be curable. But who among us has never had, or can be certain he never will have, an occasion in his life in which he has experienced some phenomenon of insanity, either an hallucination, or a profound melancholia, or a delirium? It is related that certain D'Annunzians, at the time of the occupation of Fiume, shaved their heads in order to identify themselves to some extent with their bald-headed Commandant by the 'annulment' of their hair! This fact certainly recalls one of Krafft-Ebing's patients, mentioned by Bleuler, who liked only lame women, and who could not resist the impulse to identify himself with the women he loved, by 'annulling' his own capacity to walk in the usual way. Krafft-Ebing's patient loved only the lame and could not resist his impulsive imitation; but his condition was not transitory. This is what constitutes the difference between the caprice of D'Annunzio's admirers and the psychopathology of Krafft-Ebing's patient.

The immersion of psychasthenics in the things or persons most abhorred; the metabolic deliriums of paranoia (which the French psychiatrists term late paranoia in the fourth period); delirious ideas of transformation; certain deliriums of internal possession;

lycanthropia, the Were-wolf, or Were-man, the transformations into wolves in Japan, described by Reitz ;
reptilian transformations in Russia, described by
Bechterev and so forth ; all come within the bounds of
psychiatry under the head of insane identifications.

In mental pathology we meet with other curious
symptoms, such as the delirium of negation of the whole
self—the delusion of non-existence, and that of
immortality in which, probably, the motive is also one
of identification ; but in both these cases identification
habitually involves the annulment of *both* of the factors
(*nihilism*).[19] Certain pathological conditions represent
the most exaggerated form of those transformations
of the personality or 'depersonalizations', which
are to be met with so frequently in their elementary
and temporary stages in normal individuals, which are
more accentuated and painful in the hysterio-psychas-
thenics, and finally become complete and lasting—yet less
painful, because rationalized—in victims of paranoia or
dementia præcox.[20] In cases of morbid mysticism, for
instance, the patients will support the identification by
rationalization ; thus they will calmly proclaim that they
have become God, or the Devil, or some animal, or some
powerful personage, and they actually feel themselves
divinities and rulers of the world and Nature.

Self-deification is not mysticism ; it is an insane idea,
a megalomania ; in Jung's theory it is the identification of
one's personality with that of the collective psyche.

Identifications occur, too, in certain magical performances described in the past, and in the exercises of
professional occultists of to-day—some of them in good
faith. They imply identifications so absurd that those who
accept them must either be the victims of momentary
revivals of ancient superstitions buried in the sub-

conscious, recalled by the impulses of affective exaltations, and made effective by the *will to believe* ; or else
they must be truly psychopathic, belonging to the
category either of madness or mental deficiency.   A
typical instance of magic operations by identification is
the practice of injuring a wax image of the person whom
the operator desires to harm.[21]

The identifications observed in certain mystics and
heroic converts are never pathological. They are connected
with tradition in their interpretation and are experienced
on certain occasions.   This is easily recognizable if we
consider the pathological characteristics mentioned above.
We have to remember that the two fundamental types of
post-conversional behaviour are the contemplative life,
and the social life. Now the identifications of the contemplative life, prayer and mystic union—unless they are
merely thought and felt in imitation—are exclusively
affective and temporary.   The ‘identification with
Christ ’—unless it is understood metaphorically—cannot
properly be considered, in the souls of the contemplative,
as a true process of identification ; it is merely an affective
transference of a temporary character, or only a vivid
sense of presence. The identifications of converts in
social action or charity, and of the great animators
and leaders of souls in poverty, are also simple transferences, or else elementary affective identifications, in
so far as they consist in an intense longing for identification with the poor, the sick, the outcast, or with the
external conditions of such unfortunates, followed, in
some cases, by an heroic realization of this great desire.

CHAPTER VII

THE PATHOLOGICAL THEORY IN RELIGIOUS PSYCHOLOGY

PATHOLOGICAL CONVERSIONS

FREQUENT allusions to mental pathology have been made in the foregoing chapters. The reader will recollect that senility and infirmity were considered as causes of conversion, and that mention was made of repressions, of pathological complexes, of anxiety conflicts and anxiety neuroses, of erotic mysticism, of illusions and hallucinations, of morbid projections, of 'transitivism', of rationalized affective identifications, and so forth. Since such phenomena are met with on the borderline of religion and pathology they lead to a question which must be touched on, however briefly, in order to anticipate one of the most common criticisms.

Any attempt to distinguish the normal from the pathological among religious phenomena will be wearisome, I fear, to most of my readers; but they must make a concession to the demands of professional practice, and to the mental habits of the writer. Nothing is commoner than an undervaluation of the experiences of mystics and devotees, who are often called, according to the circumstances, insane or mattoid, imbecile or hysterical, suggestible or epileptic. This habit is certainly the outcome of popular language, which does not give words the precise meaning they have for technical experts. But the practice is also common among medical alienists,

o

who in their arguments force words into channels of
diverse meanings.   To take only one example : the
'Futurists' have unceremoniously been declared
paranoiacs by two of the most eminent Italian alienists !

This chapter — it must be frankly confessed — is
suggested by my anxiety lest psychiatry, when it is
not strictly neurological (that is to say, unilateral),
continue to be a psychological-literary divagation in
bad taste.   It is high time such a state of things
ceased.   Psychiatrists should be good doctors, not
bad rhetoricians.   If psychiatry is to become a serious
medical study, it must avoid the use of inexact and
fantastic statements more or less informed by the
fashions in current philosophy, and adopt an attitude
worthier of the scientific method.

1. *Morbid Consciousness and its Diagnosis*

Twenty years ago there was probably not a single
anthropologist, physiologist, or alienist in Italy who was
not convinced that every exceptional manifestation of
human activity, whether a case of delinquency, of genius,
or of mysticism, was more or less pervaded by insanity.
From Jesus to Julian the Apostate, from St. Joan of Arc
to Napoleon, from Mahomet to Tolstoy—almost every
one of the giants of thought, feeling, or action, was
considered to be suffering from some degree of mental
alienation.[1] This extraordinary opinion found justification in two circumstances : one, that the conception of
'insanity', in consequence of the triumphs of German
and Italian psychiatry, had been immensely, though
arbitrarily, extended ; the other, that insanity had become
synonymous with the particular symptoms to be met
with in insane persons.

Of recent years things have changed, but they must

change more. To-day the insane are universally differentiated from the neuropaths, and these from the simply ' abnormal '. Abnormality is now to some extent employed in classification without any biopathological significance, but purely in the statistical sense, as is customary with the American psychopathologists, and with the school of Viola for morbid constitutions. It must, however, be added that Freudian theories have unfortunately tended to confuse afresh these differential conceptions.

This must not be taken as implying that the question, from its scientific aspect, is of easy solution. If we eliminate the sociological standpoint, to which Freudians and anti-Freudians alike appeal to-day, it is a difficult matter to define the precise terms of the antithesis between reason and madness. This is where the decisive progress of the ' somatic ' psychiatrists becomes evident, for they claim that insanity is to be defined in terms of cerebral changes. In my opinion, however, even the somatic theory, though it has sound theoretical justification, will not offer indications of use for practical purposes until it is able to furnish an exact catalogue of the somatic symptoms of insanity observable in life. This is why the psychological standpoint is continually appearing with renewed insistence in general psychiatry.

The objection to all psychological distinctions is that we find a complete series of transitions from the normal (the average temperament and character) to the abnormal or exceptional (anomalous constitutions, diatheses, neurosis, and insanity) similar to the transitions between health and disease. Nevertheless, with Meyerhof,[2] I maintain that the imperceptibility of this transition does not preclude a theoretical justification of the concept of insanity ; just as the continuity of the colours of the spectrum does not prevent our recognizing distinctions between the separate fundamental colours.

In any case, it appears to me essential to fix certain definite criteria for practical purposes; otherwise we shall be forced to continue using the terms of a psychiatric romanticism.

At the outset, it must no longer be considered justifiable to confuse the concept of ' psychic disorder ' with that of insanity. A psychic disorder, from the psychological aspect, is a variation of thought and of character in the morbid sense. It certainly goes beyond the normal degree of variation; but it is an ordinary concomitant, not only of mental alienation, but of all physical maladies and exceptional bodily states : infectious diseases, intoxications, and recurrent illnesses. It is not extraordinary that religious persons should exhibit certain symptoms of neuropsychopathy which may also be observed in cases of endocrine imbalance, or luetic disease, diabetes, gout, prostatic disease, senility, and so forth.

Insanity is an entirely different matter. Fundamentally, insanity is the antithesis of reason. In recent years Blondel has endeavoured to condense the essential character of psychoses into a formula.[3] His attempts do not appear to me to have been wholly successful, though I regard certain aspects of his exposition as of interest. His generalizations are based upon the researches and doctrines of Lévy-Bruhl, and start from the incontestable principle that man is a physical, psychical, and social entity.

Morbid consciousness appears to Blondel as a consciousness which is not socialized. According to his theory ' normal consciousness ' is everywhere permeated by collectivist elements, deriving from the social environment.

Blondel believes that the morbid consciousness is unequal to the regime of discursive and motor concepts to which normal individuals spontaneously conform. According to Blondel the 'pure psychologist' within us, which lies dormant in the subconscious of the normal social mind, awakes to consciousness in insanity. The pre-social individual re-emerges ; the psychopath is not a contemporary, or at least he finds obstacles to being one. Cœnæsthesia is distinctly individual ; it is the unassailable stronghold of the 'pure psychologist' ; it is incapable of being conceptualized. The characteristic of morbid consciousness is essentially a permanent adhesion to the 'pure psychologist', the morbid state of mind being incapable of being 'personalized'. In this way it becomes impossible for the consciousness to locate itself spontaneously in a homogeneous time. In short, the morbid consciousness is an individual consciousness incapable of transforming the 'pure psychologist' into clear and conceptualized consciousness. For Blondel, at any rate, insanity seems to be *qualitatively* distinct from the normal state.

I would not insist that Blondel's point of view can help us to determine the difference between the insane, the neuropathic, and the abnormal. And this is the precise point which we should like to have settled. We can, however, use certain of his concepts to arrive at the distinction we are looking for.

None of the most recent psychological theories of German origin, and not even the theories of Jaspers [4] and Kretschmer,[5] can provide us with any adequate instrument by which to obtain a differential conception of insanity, capable of being safely and usefully applied in medical practice. The conception of purpose- or wish-psychoses—the *Zweck-psychosen* and *Wunsch-*

psychosen, applies also to the neuroses ; it concerns itself in both cases with acute or chronic reactions of the personality to certain experiences of life—*Erlebnisse*. Psychoses and neuroses are thus regarded as maladies of the character, in other words, as the results of the actions and reactions of various conflicting forces. Thus the new 'physics of the soul' is unable to offer the differential character for which we are looking. Moreover, this point of view does not differ as much as might appear from that of psycho-analysis, for we again encounter it in Bleuler, who makes only a few distinctions and supports them merely from the social point of view.[6] To say that neuroses and psychoses are only maladjustments of the psychic life to reality is to say practically nothing.

The theory of Pierre Janet is that the neurotic never attains reality because he is an asthenic. According to Bergson, he fails to arrive because of his lack of *élan vital*. Freud regards him as possessing energy which fails because it is not rightly applied. According to Adler the neurasthenic is an inferior whose illness is a compensation. The view of modern French neurologists is that the neurotic is an invalid with a purely endogenous functioning of the affective apparatus, lacking the sustenance derived from reality ; so that everything is determined by alterations of the affective life, that is, by the general and nervous nutrition. Such theories are all useless for our purpose.

On the other hand the practical necessity of a well-defined conception of insanity and neurosis is imperative, and would obviate many existing controversies between psychopathologists and persons of culture, who are interested in the psychology of the genius, the criminal, the mystic, and the saint.

One must realize that the acceptance of a rigid concept of insanity, or of the psychoses, without also admitting the existence of transitions, might lead towards a belief in disease entities or morbid substances, which would only re-echo in a more rational form the old conception of alienation as demoniacal possession. This, of course, is far from my intention, and from what will shortly be said, it will be clear that I tend rather to deprecate the too-easy acceptance of such a pathological theory in the domain of art and religion.

There is no need to refer to Hippocrates or Wernicke, to Kräpelin or Freud, to Bleuler or Jaspers, to Blondel or Kretschmer, to outline the fundamental theory of insanity. A universal consensus exists at least upon this point : there are two essential conditions of insanity : first, that the many psychic disturbances of the individual break down his personality, which is a psychic-social synthesis, and second, that this breakdown must be more than momentary. An isolated psychic disturbance, or a sporadic appearance of morbid thought or action, does not constitute insanity. A momentary disintegration, therefore, of the psycho-social personality, such as inebriety, is not to be considered as insanity in the strictly psychiatric sense.

It is necessary that in the conduct of the subject there should be a change in the sequence of actions. In the case of insanity a rupture of mental harmony vitiates the axes of conduct, resulting in the necessity of the insane action (under the impulsion of exceptional imperatives which are always present) ; and this leads to the loss of personal autonomy. This does not mean that the madman is incapable of normal thoughts and actions, even of a very high order ; but it certainly implies that

he is *not constantly and regularly* the master of his own
conduct in harmony with social aims, but that
his life proves unharmonious in its morphology and
devious in its evolution.

There can be no doubt that insanity must be defined
in relation to time.   In fact we regard as alienation a state
of amentia which lasts for a month. We might perhaps
even consider as insanity a madness which lasted only
for a day. But we do not characterize by so serious
a term as insanity a disturbance of consciousness which
lasts for a few moments, such as a fit of convulsions, or
a fainting spell, or some such occurrence. Just in this
same way a headache which lasts only a few moments,
a rise of temperature lasting for an hour, or a single night
of insomnia, are not sufficient to constitute an illness.
And this is perfectly reasonable.   Otherwise a single
moment   of   rage,   an   instant   of   passion,   a   brief
intoxication, a rapt æsthetic contemplation, would
suffice to declare everybody insane and irresponsible.

If every deviation of our psychic personality from the
ideal middle line is to be regarded as a variation,
then a psychic disturbance is a variation which must
be considered as beyond the normal limits. Madness,
however, is the total and permanent variation of the
psychic personality.   From the psychological aspect,
the difference between normal variations and psychopathic
deviations is measurable by the quality and intensity
of the variations themselves ; but the difference between
a psychic disturbance and actual insanity is to be determined by the multiplicity and duration of the disturbance.

This view seems to me to be of capital importance,
in that it unites in a satisfactory manner the two conceptions which are fundamental to psychiatry: first,
the incurability of the judgment of the insane (which

is to be distinguished from errors of judgment) ; second, the primary or secondary diseases of the brain— destructive, inflammatory, toxic—which exist in all cases of insanity, and which are the postulate of somatic psychiatry. Hence the duration of a psychic disturbance is of particular importance ; on the one hand it leads the subject to an insane conviction or delirium ; while on the other, it enables the clinician to recognize clearly the functional alterations which lead to chemical, dynamic, or structural changes in the nervous tissue, such as are found by post-mortem examinations of the brains of mentally diseased persons. The alienists of bygone days, therefore, had reasonable grounds for affirming that insanity is always chronic, even when it is termed acute. We might go further for the sake of clearness and add to this explanation a third conception, if it were not already plainly implied in the second : which is that since every psychosis is a pathological process, it runs a necessary course. Whence it follows that it is inaccurate to speak of insanity where this is not demonstrable from the career and conduct of the individual *sub judice*.

For the last twenty-five or thirty years it has been continually re-asserted that psychiatry has entered upon its positive phase. This is certainly the case, but not merely because the cerebral processes of certain mental diseases have been discovered and elucidated. Psychiatry has become a positive science because its practitioners have now definitely discarded philosophical points of view, and firmly adhere to the postulate that every mental symptom and syndrome has its corresponding chemical and histological alterations in the nervous system, even though these may be microscopic ; and because the dissolution of the psychic personality can now be understood while the patient is alive, as being a lasting modification of the energic economy, whether psychic or nervous, even when we have not the evidence of concomitant sensory and motor symptoms ; and finally, because the modern methods of individual pyschology enable us to-day to arrive at a more precise and comprehensive descriptive and genetic analysis of the ' behaviour ' of the dement in respect of the social environment, by which means it has been possible to trace the true concatenation of the isolated symptoms of the subject's malady. The whole of modern psychiatry lies in this.

On the other hand it is short-sighted for alienists to imagine that they can solve every problem by the *post-mortem* discovery of an incontestible cerebral lesion for every psychosis—an ideal aim, as yet by no means achieved—or by substituting the genetic method for the causal in psychiatry.

Positive psychiatry does not imply psychiatry without an unknown. On the contrary, in spite of every endeavour, the medical and social estimation of what the ancients called the ' intermediate zone ' or ' borderland ' between madness and mental sanity remains extremely difficult. Particularly difficult are the transitional forms determined by the unstable criteria of social adaptation. But there does not seem, in point of fact, any justification to-day for the survival of the older sort of psychiatry.

After the pathological theory of genius and after the ' epileptoid ' theory of criminality, we have had the pathological conception of love : ' conscious obsession ', the ' amorous impulse ', the lover's anguish or satiety were the favourite arguments employed to reinforce the statement that a high proportion of criminals came from the *innamorati*. A still more recent example of such theories is the pathological theory of dreams, supported by the celebrated psychiatrist Moreau de Tours, but who is opposed on valid grounds by Freud, Vaschide, Meunier, and other psychiatrists. Among similar theories we must include the pathological theory of religion [7] which is held to-day by several psychologists, of whom Leuba is an authoritative example. This theory is made possible by the arbitrary extension of the definitions of mysticism and insanity.

Even if religion, like genius, were merely another of the fruits of insanity, it would not necessarily lose its ' value ' on that account. This is the conclusion arrived at by those who are disposed to make the largest concessions to the claims of the pathological theory. The question has received masterly treatment by William James.[8] According to this eminent psychologist, religion itself is secure, even though the morbidness of the facts of religious mysticism be admitted. As everyone knows, James argues against ' medical materialism ', establishing the distinction between *existential* judgments, and judgments of *value*. This would seem to make further argument unnecessary. If certain psychologists like Renda,[9] with whom I am in agreement, did not maintain that ' value ' is not an exclusively psychological fact, and for that reason would exclude ' value ' from the ambit of present-day scientific psychology, we should in that case find ourselves admitting, if we entrenched ourselves solely behind James's argument, that there is no distinction whatever between the mystic phenomena of religious souls and those of the insane ; and that the sole distinction—if any—would have to be sought in value or in success. This, however, appears to me to be sufficiently contestable. As a psychiatrist, I hold that semeiotic and positive mental pathology *almost invariably* offers criteria by which we can distinguish the morbid case from the individual who is not morbid, or is so only in appearance or for a momentary period.

Goethe used to say that truths are recognizable by their capacity to promote life; sterile truths, according to that standard, are not truths. This is a truly pragmatic theory. Let the theory pass, however, but the question arises: Can the affirmer and the 'realizer' of truths be insane? We must shift the inquiry from without to within, that is to say, towards the subject. In other words, we must consider whether the madman is or is not capable of recognizing the problems of life and of history, and above all, whether he is capable of arriving at their solution.

Now, it is clear that if in exceptional circumstances these problems may be grasped by one who is insane, we are not thereby justified in considering that this capacity is the result of madness. It might, perhaps, be claimed that in insanity, where the subconscious is liberated by reason of a disease of the cerebral cortex, the subject may possibly perceive and resolve such problems by the subconscious. But the insane subject, in order to perceive and to solve, that is to say, to recognize problems coming to him through the ultra-marginal obscurity, to elaborate them, and to work harmoniously, would require instruments which the automatism of the subconscious does not possess. Insanity refers to the conscious, not to the unconscious; in respect of 'dispositional' material the former may be insane and the latter sane. In a moment of unconsciousness or of automatism, an individual may perhaps make wise or original remarks; but if his consciousness is morbid he will be unable to realize them in action.

It is even probable that truly insane persons may be

indirectly of benefit to human society through good works ; but this will occur only in an age of silence or of suffering, when the people in their extremity lend ears and faith to the fleeting and obsessing invocations of an imagined saviour. But the reverse may also happen ; for instance, many great men have never succeeded, because of the unsuitability of their environment, in producing the results expected from them, for the people, having ears, do not hear. However, if such unappreciated geniuses leave works behind them, these eventually testify to the wisdom of their authors.

We need to recognize the serious difficulties of such distinctions when we are dealing with medical judgments upon individuals who have not come under direct medical observation. Even worse are opinions concerning historical personages, far removed from us in time. It is clear that in such cases the burden of proof rests with those who would sustain the theory of insanity. One testimony that Dante died of malaria is sufficient to convince us, but it would require a great many to prove that he suffered from hallucinations. And it would be necessary to have an authoritative and universal consensus of opinion to make us admit that the writer of the *Divina Comedia* was nothing more or less than a madman.

On these grounds it is evident that the science of ' historical ' psychiatry must always proceed with extreme caution and the utmost reserve, studying its cases in relation to their times, since otherwise they may be distorted beyond all measure. The social factor, indeed, can waken or re-invigorate latent germs of neurosis or madness, setting free the dormant experiences of the subconscious, as ordinarily happens in connection with revolutions, public calamities, or wars. The same thing may also happen in periods of unrest or even of apparent tranquillity, when thoughts, theories, actions, or reactions, which would be viewed as altogether morbid at other times, rise to the surface. Thus the social factor, operating on sensitive and intuitive persons, creates pseudomadness, inducing inspirations in advance of their times, which are always of social value. I recollect that at the Congress of the Italian *Società Freniatrica* held in 1899 in Naples, one of our psychiatrists made use of the term ' relatively insane ', in order to indicate those who currently pass as madmen, though in reality they are " the crystallizers of the social thought of their own epoch ". The alienist in question, Silvio Venturi, here made a valuable observation.

It is impossible to judge of the morbidness, that is, of the disproportion and inadequacy of any given reaction without knowing thoroughly the nature and conditions of the stimuli which provoked it. Thus, while it is easy to evaluate in psychiatry the conduct of an individual who is alive and present ; and while, though not so simple, it is still possible to investigate the actions of an absent contemporary concerning whom we have well-accredited documents ; it is, on the contrary, a matter of much more considerable difficulty to make just psychiatric estimates of individuals whose lives and behaviour occurred in periods remote from us. Hence it follows that historical psychiatry presupposes the historical circumstances ; and it has not merely to take into consideration the history of the individual who is to be studied and the *general* history of the country and the epoch to which that personage belonged, but also the *particular* history of the period and locality in which the individual lived and worked.

Many people attach considerable importance to the

opinions of contemporaries who believed in the madness of historical figures. This is to re-echo the adage that the voice of the people is the voice of God. Undoubtedly a contemporary verdict of insanity possesses a certain degree of value. There are, nevertheless, many matters to be sifted. In the first place, we have to consider whether the conception of insanity of that period was identical with the conception of insanity at the present time. In the second place, were the contemporary judges of those days possessed of a knowledge and culture equalling that of present day judges of sanity and madness ? Were they competent to distinguish from the insane those who were suffering merely from neuroses and other con- stitutional derangements ? And lastly, were such opinions the judgments of many ? Did they meet with general acceptance ? Have they been invalidated by the lapse of time and the change of place ? All of these are arduous considerations indeed.

When a psychosis was obviously due to a disease of the brain, a diagnosis may be possible to-day. But when the disease itself was not visible, and the case was merely one of some ' anomaly ' of behaviour, judgment becomes radically invalidated. Let us take simply ' abnormal ' individuals at a distance of centuries and in situations remote from us, and ask ourselves whether the evaluation of their cases by modern psychiatrists can be considered seriously. At the very outset' there is the objection that such judges are ignorant or quasi-ignorant of history, or at best have but a modicum of knowledge, insufficient to criticize the sources of information or to sift the admissibility of evidence and opinion.

The crudest example of this ineptitude is that of the author of the *Folie de Jésus*, who bases his diagnosis exclusively upon the authority of the accounts of the

Evangelists, there being no other sources! The "*ex ore
tuo te judico*" is in this case an impudent sophistry, for
if Christ's conduct was that of a madman, the
Evangelists who recounted it, and the millions of persons
—cultured and uncultured alike—who have read and
believed their accounts, would easily have discovered the
facts, since in every age historians and men of culture
have invariably made distinctions between madness and
mental sanity. To base a theory on certain phrases or
on the isolated commentary of contemporaries, then, can
only be regarded as a form of misplaced ingenuity.

Some psychiatrists think they have indisputable
proofs of the madness of St. Francis of Assisi, in the
opinions of his contemporaries.[10] The *Fioretti* may admit
that St. Francis was regarded as foolish, and that "like
a madman he was scoffed at and pelted with stones and
with mud by his relatives and by strangers". But there
is something more to observe here. It is quite common
to hear in connection with exceptional persons that they
have the reputation of being 'fools'. The populace did not
consider only St. Francis as mad, but also Brother Egidio,
Brother Bernard, and others of the friars whom he sent
out upon missions to Germany and Hungary. Indeed all
who ran counter to the currently accepted levels of morals
and habits were so accounted. It is, however, to be noted
that the multitude in former centuries, as at the present
day, has never attached the same meaning to the terms
'madman' or 'fool' that is attached to them in psychopathology. It is certainly true that even in our own
times the term 'madman' is still gratuitously applied
to the greatest poets and philosophers, and to the most
distinguished artists and politicians. Great national and
international movements, inspired by the loftiest social
interests, have been looked upon as classic instances of

psychopathic epidemics. But this is merely an ignorant extension of the term. For the rest, the most modern school of psycho-pathologists—to take Jaspers as one instance—declares that the word 'madman' is devoid of significance, since it can indicate equally an idiot or a man of genius.

St. Francis did undoubtedly commit extravagant acts, but aside from the fact that it is difficult for us now to estimate them in their true proportions, they did not constitute any serious evidence in support of madness, even for his own contemporaries. Tertullian, too, was considered to have been a 'cracked brain' at times, because of the extraordinary fashion of his attire after his conversion to Christianity. This, however, did not lead his contemporaries to regard him as a true madman ; nor has any alienist—unless, perhaps, we except those of to-day—discovered any insanity in this intellectual Carthaginian.

Any reputation of madness in regard to St. Francis of Assisi certainly must have vanished by 1310, when Dante mentioned him in the famous passage of the *Paradiso*. In addition to this, it is undisputed that, when immediately following the death of St. Francis, Gregory IX summoned the College of Cardinals to discuss the reasons for his canonization, no mention was then made of madness. Nor did any word of it circulate on the occasion when the canonization was promulgated at Assisi, although only a short time intervened between his death and this occurrence, on 16th July, 1228. Then, too, the extreme rapidity of the diffusion of the Franciscan order—which spread throughout the whole of Europe—would seem to be an argument against the existence of any public opinion that St. Francis was a madman. According to Pier delle Vigne, the chancellor of the Emperor Frederick,

P

one half of Christendom joined the Third Order of St. Francis and " because of that diffusion the power of Heaven became far more formidable, more profitable than that of Earth ".[11]

Besides this lack of objective proofs, an important pragmatic question arises : Could a madman be so altruistic, so flawless in morals, so prodigious in organization, as to maintain his activity throughout a period of at least twenty years (the period of time that elapsed between his conversion and his death) without developing dementia ? This, of course, is the objection of positive psychiatry.

Consequently we must agree that before having recourse to equivocal, fallacious, or extrinsic criteria, it is essential to prove a case with the sound methods of positive psychiatry, based upon facts belonging to the present, or facts brought up to date by an historical criticism which is above suspicion.

The evidence of facts and their careful examination lead us to distinguish between ' normal ' and ' pathological ' mysticism.

2. Normal, Impure, and Morbid Mysticism : Pathological Conversions

Everyone knows what is meant by ' normal ' mysticism. It antedates every positive religion. Mysticism, indeed, means simply the contact of our ego with everything that seems to us highest, most unattainable, most mysterious. The experiences of mysticism, indeed, transcend all religions and are the common heritage of all sensitive and receptive souls. Since empirical psychology finds irrational intuition and emotion among the psychic functions along with reason, and since, on the other hand, general psychology need not confine itself to the testimony of arid souls and sluggish brains any more than to the statements of members of an anti-clerical assembly, mysticism may therefore be considered entirely normal.

Owing to the considerable extension given to the term, the public think they can designate mysticism and asceticism and similar phenomena of consciousness ' à l'état fort ', as nothing more nor less than *alienations of the mind*.[12] Ribot,[13] however, has already dissipated certain misconceptions, and we can re-affirm the fact that alienation—if it exists—occurs only in the case of a lasting *état fort*, with its inevitable impairment of the psychic personality and the organism of the patient.

Nothing whatever is gained by returning to the arguments of medical polemics in support of the patho-logical theory of mysticism. Mysticism is not counter to reason ; it is beyond it. Reason is discursive ; but beyond the ' socialized ' consciousness there exists the individual consciousness, which completes the other, or—what amounts to the same thing—is the mould in which the social consciousness is shaped. Contact with mystery does not, in fact, disturb the scientific consciousness, because there is no mystery in science. Mystery is beyond and above what we know and what we imagine ourselves capable of knowing. It is not the function of logic to effect the connection between things and their meanings, hidden in symbols. It is the function of intuition, of poetry, of life.

Mystic analytic knowledge is, again, a different matter ; it consists in the intellectual-verbal translation of that which in reality possesses no precise imagery, which has no adequate expression, unless perhaps, as Goethe thought, in music. But it is not justifiable to regard such mysticism as the exceptional state of consciousness which we call morbid. The intellectualizing of our emotions is a normal process. One might, perhaps, consider that the immersion of self in the mystic world of fantasy, with its strange arabesques, its exotic and instable legends and mythology, is the sign of a morbid consciousness. We must not equivocate on this point; such mysticism may be poetry, or at the utmost the superstructure of a more or less æsthetic faith; but it cannot be insanity unless the world of fantasy is intensely and permanently conceived of as a tangible reality because of the aims and necessities inherent in the individual enslaved by his cœnæsthesia (according to Blondel) and deaf to the collective voice, unless, in short, the world is translated into a personal and illogical conception.

To give an example : in mysticism there is a frequently mentioned 'law of substitution' (Huysmans, in his *En Route*, repeatedly alludes to 'substitution by prayer') by which the mystic deliberately takes upon himself the burden of a terrible struggle against strong temptation, intentionally 'substituting' himself for an individual who, in such a conflict against evil, would be unable to exert an equal degree of resistance. In this case there is a fusion of a profound faith and an altruism which is heroic. It is self-evident that a 'symptom' of this kind does not belong to psychiatric semeiotics.

The traditional mysticism of the positive religions and that of devout souls is not to be regarded as morbid, precisely because it is not a *personal* production, the work, that is, of the 'pure psychologist' within the individual, and thus does not invest the whole psycho-social personality of the subject, but leaves his recognition of social and cosmic reality unaltered. The mysticism of Dante and of all the great philosophers and saints and poets should be considered as normal, although accompanied by dreams and visions, by revelations and intuitions, by moral fevers and by the most daring symbolism. For example, 'the religion of the heart' to which Dante refers in the *Convivio* was combined in him with the most rigorous sense of rationality, thus forming a great and pure consciousness, free from all traces of morbidity.

On the other hand, morbid mysticism—which in its ultimate analysis proves to be a pseudo-mysticism or as Récéjac characterizes it a *degradation of mysticism*—both in process of formation, and in its final form, is entirely personal, that is to say, extraneous to any ethico-social imperative. It is this extraneousness which appears to me as constituting, from the psychological aspect, the most specific mark of morbidness. Morbidness may, however, arise in other conditions ; for instance, by an unwonted intensity and frequency in an individual of traditional mystic phenomena, in themselves normal ; or by their occurrence in subjects who are already mentally diseased.

Experience teaches us that it is by no means exceptional for devout souls—even those in no way diseased—to undergo mystic crises containing a strongly erotic element, more or less voluntarily combated and repressed. Such cases, however, are not true instances of morbid mysticism, chiefly because the psychic personality of the patient is not subjugated in any lasting way ; but on the other hand, we cannot regard such cases as corresponding to the normal mysticism of tradition. This is why in practice there is a third classification of mysticism, which is termed ' impure '. ' Impure ' mysticism, as contrasted with the normal, which we call 'pure', is so called because it does not appear in the subject with that degree of sublimation which 'pure' mysticism has reached in the evolution of individual and social ethics. 'Impure' mysticism is atavistic—a throw-back to the roots of the individual; a momentary regression to origins. On the other hand, 'morbid' mysticism, in the psychopathic sense, is not only morbid on account of its origins, but also by reason of the mental states of the mystic, which will neither allow a voluntary sublimation nor the acceptance of traditional religious experience, which has been already sublimated (by definition). Finally, morbid mysticism does not allow of the recognition of its own inferiority.

As everyone knows, an individual may experience sexual emotions while undergoing mystic experiences; which confirms the affinity of origin of these two affective states. This fact, however, does not give the slightest character of abnormality to the mystic experience itself. Havelock Ellis, who is under no suspicion of partiality in this relation, states that " a man who is carried away by religious emotion cannot be held responsible for the indirect emotional results of his condition, but he is responsible for their control ".[14]

This is very true; the fact of a common origin is insufficient to establish a pathological connection between mysticism and eroticism. The relation needs to be verified not only in the unconscious and in automatism but in the consciousness of the individual. This is why there is little support for the pathological theory of mysticism in the fact that eroticism and mysticism have been found in association throughout the history of all religions and customs.

Religious prostitution—described by Herodotus and Strabo—which was so common in Cyprus and in Phœnicia,

Carthage, Judea, Armenia, India, and elsewhere, and not infrequently associated with cruelty of every kind and even with human sacrifice, is only an additional proof of the community or affinity of sex and religion, which we have already emphasized. But this does not justify the belief that these prostitutes and sanguinary sacerdotalists were all insane and on a par with our own paranoiacs, epileptics, and psychopathic erotics. Tradition, custom, adaptation, and imitation sufficiently explain the practices of ancient religions and the aberrations of Asiatic cults transported to Rome, such as those of Cybele and Attis.[15]

Such distinctions are indispensable if we are to avoid obscure and equivocal misunderstandings which confound the truth, and which have been constantly employed by the polemicist, the dilettante, and the pedant.

A digression must here be made on the subject of the community or affinity of the origins of religious emotion and sexual emotion, in order to avoid misconception. The psychologist and positivist philosopher, Ribot,[16] clearly states that : " La psychologie des auteurs, qui réduisent tout (la religion) à un érotisme dévié, est beaucoup trop simpliste et nullement applicable à tous les cas." The psychiatrist and rationalist sociologist, Forel, who has been so largely occupied with this problem, observes : " It would be absolutely false to attempt to affirm that religion in itself is derived from sexual sensations." [17]

These two quotations, selected at random from a number, clearly indicate that, for the positivists, this community and affinity (or, to be more precise, direct derivation) refer, not to all religious experiences, but only to such as provoke a personal enjoyment in the subject ; a gratification which he does not project upon his neighbour, or upon humanity as a whole.

When Schopenhauer in his work *Neue Paralipomena* dwelt on the similarity between certain creations of genius and certain forms of the masculine sexual instinct, and when he declared that "love is the burning point of the will", he enunciated nothing new, and offered no proof of the pathology of genius. When ethnologists, and physicians like Forel and Bloch, and many others point to the connection between sexuality and religion, they merely repeat a conviction that has been widely diffused since the Middle Ages. The unfortunate thing is that one cannot derive from these facts the practical deductions which so many would like. Therefore there is nothing surprising to me—or to any who interest themselves in questions of science, apart from politics—· in the statement of the highly competent and non-Catholic Ivan Bloch : " It is incorrect and irrational to reproach the Catholic Church, as some modern writers have done —though they are certainly not writers highly versed in the history of civilization—for the presence and the influence of elements of sexuality in its dogmas and rituals." [18]

In closing this digression, we would re-emphasize, in deference to the facts, that it is essential to distinguish pathological from normal mysticism, and to divide the latter into ' impure ' and ' pure ' (normally sublimated) mysticism. It is the pathological subject who displays repulsive monstrosities, or at least an almost systematic mixture of mystic symptoms with symptoms of eroticism and insanity.

The literature of psychiatry is full of facts which

demonstrate the frequency with which mysticism is associated with sexuality in the insane. Esquirol, Icard, Friedreich, Schroeder van der Kolk, Krafft-Ebing, and among later writers, Lombroso, Murisier, Roemer, Karl Holl, Hermann Gunkel, Forel, Heinrich Weinel, Bloch, and Havelock Ellis have all expounded and commented upon cases of this description. Mystic-erotic aberrations have been found also among the great mystics of history. In Jakob Boehme, for example, we find the identification with Christ, which, in the sense we have already explained, is common to all mystics ; but he had also a strange conception of Lucifer and Adam, which had a basis in homosexual and hermaphroditic tendencies, with numerous paranoidal symptoms.[19]

Erotic mysticism has predominated in certain environments in every age and in all places. A modern example full of tragedy is that of Rasputin.[20] There are also individual instances of exaltation which are very close to the morbid, such as Fra Bianco da Siena, and Jacopone da Todi. These cases are partly attributable to their epoch, and to the customs of their day, and partly, one cannot doubt, to the ardour of their own temperament. The ' scatophagous ' mystics, who are not uncommon, as the Catholic writer Maxime de Montmorand himself has candidly avowed, do not always deserve to be considered madmen, although scatophagy is habitually seen among idiots and dements. *L'histoire saintement sordide* of Sister Louise du Néant, which is alluded to by Brémond, does not constitute the typical history of all mystics, however overcome by the passion of humility. We must not forget that Sister Louise had lived in a hospital for the insane !

On the other hand, the recognition of transitional zones is here relevant, since the conception of normality is extremely elastic, and there is a great multiplicity of individual variants from type.

Oskar Pfister [21] recently enumerated the symptoms of morbid mysticism, both physiological and psychic, in connection with the study of a mediæval nun, called Marguerite Ebner. Among the symptoms dealt with were the identification of herself with Christ, the projection of her own sensuality upon Christ, the polarization of antagonistic tendencies, and so forth. But Pfister very rightly emphasizes the fact that Marguerite Ebner's was not a true sublimation, but at most an uplifting of the libido towards transformation into higher activity of ethical value.

It is indeed true that certain conversions are arrested at the first phase of sublimation. Others, even more common, never attain even that phase of sublimation, but indulge in a purely theoretical sublimation, while in practice Eros overcomes Caritas, or else the former celebrates a fleeting and monstrous alliance with the latter. But such bankruptcies of conversion do not count. In true converts, with whom we are here concerned, the conversional cycle is completed. In them, the process of conversion finds its outlet in action and in a new will to live.

If we pass into the purely psychiatric field, the element of pathology is enormously increased. How many cases there are of psychopathic hysteria, of paraphrenia, of epilepsy, and of paranoia, which present to us ecstatic phenomena, sensory hallucinations with an erotic religious content, kinæsthetic, verbomotor, or genital hallucinations, plans for grandiose ecclesiastical or social reforms with a sexual basis, prophecy during sexual excitement, and the like. These are cases of true pathological mysticism, that is, of the rebirth of the mystic subconscious and its deformation in some personalities, due to abnormalities or disease (primary or secondary) of the cerebral cortex. The psychosis itself, however, consists precisely in this abnormality or disease, which eventually expresses itself in terms of consciousness, and in the expression deforms the sub-conscious material; it does not consist in the liberated and re-activated subconscious material itself, or in the symptoms considered by themselves. An hallucination alone, a crisis of dysthymia, lipothymy, stigmatization, the products of the deepest stratum of the subconscious, are insufficient to characterize a person as insane, or to characterize him as religious. What is further needed is the conscious elaboration of the contents which have been liberated.

Finally, we are justified in inquiring whether or no there are distinctly morbid conversions. There can be no doubt whatever that such cases are to be met with—and indeed with some frequency—during the so-called epidemics of mysticism. In these cases the morbidity is demonstrable, less by the manner in which they are determined—through suggestion, imitation, or fear—than by excess in mystic practices and the concomitance of facts which are undoubtedly morbid. That these are cases of pseudo-conversion is demonstrated by their transience.

Individual morbid conversions are much less common than morbid mass conversions. I have, however, had the opportunity, during the past few years, of observing two cases of women suffering from a manic-depressive psychosis. One, a Protestant, and the other, a Jewess, had become fervent converts to Catholicism, during the phase of depression. I have no history of the former after her conversion. As to the other, I know that at the end of the depressive cycle she still remained a Christian, but all the fervour had burnt itself out, and with it, the beginning of her sublimation of the libido.

More interesting still is the case of another of my patients, also affected by a manic-depressive psychosis of the classic type, although the symptoms were not always serious. During the manic phases of the psychosis, this patient passed from Catholicism to Anglicanism, and from Anglicanism again to other forms of religion, making these changes of cult several times, and on one occasion with public ceremony. In this lady's case, however, there was a total absence of sublimation. From that aspect, therefore, this case must be considered a pseudo-conversion, even if it cannot be called morbid.

Morbid conversions are to be met with in art. For my own part, I cannot but believe that the conversion of Madame Gervaisais, the heroine of the celebrated novel by the brothers de Goncourt was of the morbid type.[22] It does not matter whether or no its morbid nature was recognized as such even by the authors.

3. *Visions, Voices, Revelations, and Hallucinations in Mystics and in the Insane*

Nothing is more common in the legends of the saints, and the histories of the converted, than their belief in sensory contact with the divine. Following the vision of Damascus, similar phenomena of communication between God and the elect were multiplied. After St. Francis received the stigmata, there followed a succession of some forty other stigmatizations. And now we must ask ourselves whether these followers of St. Francis and all the visionaries of history should rightly be considered as mentally affected ? No. On the contrary, we consider that an advanced semeiotic can offer criteria, at least in certain cases, for distinguishing the isolated phenomena which many religious souls present from those similar or indeed analogous symptoms displayed by the insane.

It is a serious mistake to transfer to the field of normal individual psychology, conceptions, interpretations, and terminology properly belonging to psychopathology. At one period the term ' degeneration ' was thus abused ; a little later we heard of ' double personalities ' ; and more recently still of the ' pathological unconscious '.

I think that a greater degree of caution in argument and a more penetrating observation and analysis, would materially aid in clarifying the situation. For example, among the younger psychiatrists the terms *hysterico-psychopathic* or *epileptic* are gratuitously applied to every religious mystic who is reported to have had experience of states of ecstasy with visions or crises of a like nature. They forget that the true hysterical ecstasy, somnambulism or vigilambulism, and the equivalent psycho-epilepsy, are all phenomena followed by amnesia. When the saints or the mystics present phenomena of apparent ecstasy or rapture, accompanied by complete cutaneous anæsthesia and followed by amnesia, the physician cannot fail to recognize the morbid character of these symptoms. But the truth is that in the majority of instances, even when insensibility accompanies the state of rapture, there is no amnesia, and whatever occurs in these ecstasies is remembered by the subjects themselves. In such cases no psychiatrist can diagnose such raptures as somnambulistic or epileptic attacks.

Jœrgensen has written that Christianity is a religion of revelations and of visions, meaning by revelations what others call inspirations, that is to say, certain ideas or decisions inspired in the subject by the divinity revealing itself in this express way.[23] It is necessary to determine what is meant, in mysticism, by *visions*.

Let us begin by observing that such a definition is no easy one, because of the inaccurate and tendential manner in which visions are described. One is justified, moreover, in observing that true hallucinations in the psychiatric sense, are very much rarer among mystics than is commonly thought. Even the vision of Damascus, related in the Acts of the Apostles, was probably not altogether a true hallucination. Saul saw a flash of light streaming from heaven. The Christophany and the voice heard could have been phenomena of another nature, provoked by the initial sensory phenomenon. We know that the Messianic or apostolic conscience always had formative elements other than sensorial factors, to which, however, their formation was often referred. Thus the Christophanies of the apostles and the disciples were assuredly not true hallucinations, or, at any rate, they were not hallucinations alone. The Acts say in one passage that the companions of Saul heard the voice but saw nothing; while in another, that they saw the light but heard no voice. The last version would seem to be the more probable. The words of Jesus in Aramaic, referred to in the Acts, are considered by many as an oratorical fabrication interpolated into Paul's self-defence before Agrippa. Thus it seems probable that the pathological feature was the blinding of his sight, and not the vision and the voices. Nor can the subsequent interpretations of his vision given by Paul himself be regarded as pathological.

It is necessary to go deeply into this most important problem of mystic visions. St. Paul ascended into the third heaven, as Dante visited the three other-worldly

realms ; Christ spoke through St. Catherine of Siena, as
Zarathustra through Nietzsche (this is the simile of
Jœrgensen). Certain visions of St. Catherine of Siena and
of St. Bridget, like those of the mystics Suzo and
Swedenborg, are phenomena very similar to the visions of
poets, and of artists in general. We shall see later wherein
lies the difference. We must meanwhile limit ourselves to
the statement of a serious doubt as to the possibility of
a psychiatric explanation of mystic visions. The diagnoses
of epileptic or hysterical hallucination advanced by
certain psychiatrists are totally unjustifiable, even when
they do not follow the deplorable practice of exaggerating
the clinical picture whenever a given case fails to present
the necessary features, an easy method of certain alienists,
fortunately of a former day.

The visions and revelations of the mystics and the
devout have no specific characteristic other than the
'state of faith' by which they are accompanied, that is,
the interpretation of their causation and their content.
Fantasy plus faith ; that is the substance of the greater
part of mystic visions and voices. Faith certainly does
not admit of a psychiatric explanation, inasmuch as faith
and belief are states of the most normal consciousness,
closely studied by contemporary psychology. An
individual who refers something exceptional which has
befallen his body or mind to the transcendental, is not to
be regarded as mentally affected on that account, any
more than the traditionalist, the imitator, the illiterate, or
the ingenuous child ; nor must we confuse with the
psychopath the subject who is impelled by moral impulses
to return towards the faith of his childhood.

It is an undoubted fact, and one which many authors
frequently confirm, that fantasy-vision, rather than true
hallucination,[24] characterizes religious spirits. If we

read attentively we find frequent evidence of the individual himself being clearly conscious that he is not concerned with an experience of sensory reality, but simply with a vision, the content of which he accepts. We read of just such an instance in the Acts of the Apostles, when we come to the account of St. Peter in prison. To him, confined in chains, there appeared an angel who unloosed him, and then Peter " went out, and followed him ; and wist not that it was true which was done by the angel ; but thought he saw a vision." (Acts XII, 9.)

At the time of the celebrated conversion of Ratisbonne and again on the occasion of the fiftieth anniversary of that event in 1892, the convert was alluded to as insane, particularly on account of his vision of the Immaculate Virgin which he had had in the church of Sant' Andrea delle Fratte in Rome.[25] But perusal of the life of Ratisbonne, who survived his conversion by more than forty-two years—he died at the age of seventy in 1884—and the critical study of his works, sufficiently refute all diagnosis of mental infirmity. As to the vision, which was said to be the cause of his unlooked-for conversion, a careful analysis enables us to infer that it was nothing else but a most luminous, clear, and lively reproduction of the already vivid image of the Madonna stamped on a medal which he had been wearing round his neck for several days. Ratisbonne was never subject to hallucinations before or after the vision in Sant' Andrea delle Fratte. But the state of his soul during those days of spiritual ferment, would alone supply sufficient reason for the vision.

Many writers have declared that the great mystics of history were almost invariably subject to hallucinations. We now know how to estimate the value of such sweeping statements. At the same time we must admit that the reliable biographies we possess—not the legendary lives compiled for the edification of the faithful—and the autobiographies of the mystics themselves (when these are not purely oneiric or fantastic productions) do indeed reveal *pseudo-hallucinations* (psychic hallucinations), or rudimentary hallucinations (elementary or abortive hallucinations). For instance Swedenborg [26] for the most part did not experience psycho-sensory phenomena, but usually had elementary visions or auditions—which were even ' willed '—when he concentrated upon a particular point, whether exterior or interior.

Hence it is perfectly natural that a minor sensory event (a rudimentary hallucination) or a mere excited imagination should provoke the apparition of a content, already conscious or unconscious, which reproduces the dominant ideas of the subject and his most powerful aspirations. Such phenomena are ' wish-fulfilments ', akin to the realizations of desires which occur in dreams. At this point, the vision or the audition becomes complex, and takes on the appearance of a plastic hallucination.

The greater part of the ' wonderful visions ' of the Blessed Angela of Foligno were visions of the inner sight. And in the same way the ' divine embrace ' and the miraculous visions of the Body of Jesus Christ and of the Infant Jesus were nothing but ' elevations in spirit '.

All this occurs also in the insane, as well as in the hallucinated. The difference here is that the insane are chronic patients (affected with dissociation or with mental disintegration), such as the paranoids, the paraphrenics, and imbeciles in the delirious phase; and their recognition is an easy matter for the competent psychiatrist.

Delacroix [27] has made a conscientious and extremely accurate study of the hallucinatory phenomena of the mystics. He is also of opinion that these phenomena are almost never sensory visions or external auditions; in other words they are not true hallucinations of sight or hearing. All the mystics distinguish between ' external ' and ' internal ' voices, between ' true ' visions and ' fantastic ', and distinguish both these from the words and visions ' of the intellect '. And indeed each of these is an entirely different phenomenon. Suzo, for example, usually had visions like dreams with the eyes open; but not oneiric hallucinations such as are described by the psychiatrist Régis. In the mystics we are dealing with the occurrence of phenomena resembling mental representations, accompanied by the sense of passivity (imposed from without, or, in other words, by God).

These phenomena have been called ' psychic hallucinations ' by Baillarger, and ' pseudo-hallucinations ' by Hagen. Delacroix, however, has some interesting remarks to make about them. Baillarger [28] bases his category of psychic hallucinations on the testimony of the mystics, on the observation of dreams, as well as on the study of the insane. Séglas,[29] who has made a brilliant study of the question, concludes that the psychic hallucinations of Baillarger are not all of one kind, but in reality include : (1) simple reveries of the waking state ; (2) mental representations which are vivid, precise, automatic, and not produced at will (the pseudo-hallucinations of Kandisky) ; (3) psycho-motor (verbal) hallucinations.

Those belonging to the second category are most frequently described by the mystics who allude to them as " visions with the eyes of the soul ", and so forth. It is to be regretted that Séglas should have admitted the second category of psychic hallucinations, not because they occur frequently in the insane, but simply on the basis of the evidence of the mystics and that of Baillarger and of Kandisky ! As is well known, the latter described in 1885 two cases of pseudo-hallucination. The first was a case of visual representations of great intensity which were involuntary and which occurred with closed eyes. In the second, the patient interpreted his visual and auditory pseudo-hallucinations as persecution ; he imagined that it was his enemies who compelled him to hear and to see with the ears and the eyes of the spirit, and not with his bodily eyes and ears. It is clear that insanity is discernible only in the second of these cases, and that the madness consisted in the nature of the patient's interpretations of his hallucinations. According to Kandisky pseudo-hallucination is something half-way between sensory hallucination and mental representation, and, taken alone, does not imply alienation.

We conclude, then, that some forms of hallucinatory phenomena—with the exception of sensory hallucinations —are not to be found among the specific symptoms of insanity, but are rather to be met with among the mystics, as we learn from their own direct testimony ; and other forms are peculiar, not to the insane, but to normal persons of extreme sensibility. The *hallucination of presence*, the ' sense of presence ', that is, the certainty of the presence of a person who cannot be perceived by any of the senses, is a common species of hallucination of the muscular sense, which many observers, myself included, have discovered in perfectly normal individuals, in no other way subject to hallucinations. St. Theresa declared : " The soul sees clearly that someone is present, even though he is not perceptible under any form." It is to be noted that the saint uses the word ' sees ' not ' feels ' : this excludes the factor of tactile kinæsthesia.

A Jewish convert, of complete mental sanity, whose confessions are to be found in Father Mainage's volume, *Nos Convertis*, expresses herself in the following words : " One evening I felt the presence of my mother. Nothing was to be seen or heard through the normal channels. Yet I had the strongest and the most convincing certainty that I had perceived *something*, through I know not what unknown sense." And one could multiply similar quotations.

The sense of presence, according to Delacroix and many others, is not inherently pathological, but is rather to be considered as a dream-phenomenon. I have, in fact, observed it in the hypnagogic state in completely normal subjects, intelligent and sensitive. I would even go further and say that the sense of presence can be experimentally induced. By concentrating her attention and desires on the memory of a loved person, who may be dead or at a distance, a lady of my acquaintance (of absolute mental sanity and balance) can succeed in producing in herself the impression that that person is ' near '.

We next come to examine what modern psychiatrists have to say upon the subject of pseudo-hallucinations, and I can find nothing to contradict what has already been said. The pseudo-hallucinations which occur are chiefly auditory ; occasionally visual instances are also found. Bleuler describes some which he has called ' extracampal ', because the subject sees the hallucination, but beyond the range of his visual field, at its extreme edge, or behind his back.

According to Kräpelin these phenomena are merely intensely vivid representations or abortive sensory hallucinations—' rudimentary hallucinations ' as I called them just now. Lugaro,[30] on the contrary, regards them as mental representations, identical with the normal processes of thought, provoked by cerebral stimuli in the representational centres, but isolated and detached from the ordinary processes of association, and therefore regarded as objective by the subject. From what Tanzi and Lugaro say, it would appear that their morbid character is derived from the interpretations which the patients give to them, and from the symptoms by which they are accompanied, such as true hallucinations, impulses corresponding to the content of the pseudo-hallucination, impulses which are altogether automatic, a subsequent more or less complete amnesia, disturbance of character, and more especially, dissociation of thought. If pseudo-hallucinations are said to be specific to paranoid dementia it is for the precise reason that they are an immediate associative effect of the disturbance of the will which is so characteristic of these chronic patients. When they are observed in subjects free from schizophrenia, that is to say persons who are not dissociated, we cannot regard them as being definite symptoms of insanity. That the mystics with psychic hallucinations are not schizophrenes is clearly demonstrated by the unity of their thought and of their conduct, by the presence of complete and frequent volitional processes, and also by the noticeable absence of the classic symptoms of schizophrenic dissociation. For example, in the histories of the mystics and in the souls of the religious and the devout, I have never discovered symptoms of insane negativism—neither ideas of negation (however abundant the phenomena of psychic conflict), nor what Bleuler [31] calls symptoms of ' autismus '.

There remain the true and complete hallucinations. One cannot deny that these may at times be found among mystics. But it is well known that true hallucinations—

that is to say, hallucinations accompanied by a maximum
of sensory experience—do not constitute actual alienation.
Everyone recognizes that hallucinations, and not illusions
alone, are possible occurrences in moments of altered
nervous and psychic tension, such as general hypotension
and hypotonia, resulting from fasting and exhaustion.
This has been observed by all the older alienists, and,
among Italians, notably by Lombroso. Experiencing
hallucinations, therefore, means nothing more serious
than finding oneself in an exceptional state of nervous
tension. This accounts for the fact that Professor Henry
Sidgwick was able to find, as the result of his famous
inquiry, that seven and eight-tenths per cent of the
men, and twelve per cent of the women questioned, had
had hallucinations.

The difference between the hallucinations of the sane
and those of the insane, consists in this—that while they
are uncritically accepted by the latter, the sane rectify
them.   Goethe and Verga experienced hallucinations,
which they corrected. Not so the paralytic dement, Guy
de Maupassant. If, however, the sane subject is already
in the religious ' state of faith ', he will accept the content
of the hallucination, and will not rectify the hallucination
itself, since its morbid mechanism escapes his recognition,
and—because of his faith—he will even believe his vision
possible. Such a mystic might certainly merit the title
of dreamer or visionary, and come, eventually, to be called
hallucinated ; but never, unless other facts bear it out,
could he be called a madman.

Indeed, if one considers the great controversies which
have always raged about the subject of hallucinatory
phenomena (psychiatrists should re-read the celebrated
discussion of the Société Médico-psychologique of Paris
in 1856, in which the most famous psychiatrists of that

classic epoch in French psychiatry took part), if one studies the discussion carried on to-day in regard to psychic hallucinations, one becomes more and more persuaded of the truth of what was said above—that even true sensory hallucinations are compatible with a sound mentality. This was the claim of the French alienists, particularly Parchappe, in times past, and in our day of Schüle and almost all psychiatrists. One is persuaded that a true hallucination once experienced may be recalled by an effort of the will, as the great alienist Brierre de Boismont demonstrated; and, finally, that insanity does not consist in any particular symptom, but in a *disturbance of the entire psychic personality*, which produces the mental compulsion which is the true characteristic of mental disease.

I may mention one further fact, which, in my opinion, can be utilized for a definitive differential diagnosis between normal and pathological mysticism.

If mystics subject to sensory or psychic hallucinations were mentally diseased they would—at least with the passage of years—fall into dissociation of the schizophrene type. In fact, all alienists, and especially Bianchi in Italy, agree that the frequency of hallucinations and the long duration of the hallucinatory periods lead to disintegration of the psychic personality, and thus to a state of permanent and incurable mental deficiency. Now if, as we know, there are mystics concerning whom it is recorded that throughout their whole lives they had visions, hallucinatory auditions, the sense of presence, voices of the soul, and so forth—and examples of such mystics are numerous—who, nevertheless, have not ended in dementia, we are forced to come to one or the other of two possible conclusions: either that their real or presumptive hallucinations were not truly of the kind which the insane

present, or else that notwithstanding their hallucinations, their mental and moral constitutions were extraordinarily resistant.

In conclusion, the individual symptoms of psychopathology are of value in so far as they are indications of
an insane ' behaviour ' determined by a lasting alteration
of the entire personality of the patient. The course of
insanity differs entirely from the normal course of
sanctity, even in cases which are characterized by the
occurrence of solemn mystic phenomena, such as visions,
ecstatic crises, stigmata, and so on.

After a study of the entire personality and an accurate
analysis of the biography of St. Paul, no psychiatrist
could confuse him with Brandano, ' Christ's Madman '.
Although St. Paul was a man of weak constitution, timid
and passionate, and possibly an epileptic, he journeyed
without ceasing under the impulse of a powerful idealism,
preaching, teaching, writing, arguing, exposing himself
to grave dangers, and in the end facing martyrdom.
Brandano lived between 1490 and 1554. At the age of
thirty-eight he became suddenly converted after receiving
an injury to one of his eyes ; but he continued to behave
with impulsiveness, pride, and hatred, even daring to make
an attempt upon the life of Don Diego de Mendoza ; and
died equally without infamy or fame, a little before the
fall of the Republic of Siena for whose sake he had so
constantly struggled and prophesied.[32] So, again, there
is no parallel between the Messianism of Jesus and that
of the many other messiahs who have preceded and
followed him down to the time of the pseudo-Delphic
Naundorff [33] or the still more recent David Lazzaretti.[34]
The messianic and reformative ideas of certain unstable
minds may, indeed, contain great truths and lofty ideals,

but the analysis and history of such individuals make it easy to distinguish the doctrines from those who profess them. No chronic madman who uttered prophecies analogous to those of Brandano could be compared with the prophets of Israel, though they also were rebellious souls, violent and exalted by the calamities of their country and aspirations for its advancement.

In the same way, the plainly pathological identifications with Christ or the Apostles of the famous Clystowtzy Russians, cannot in any way be likened to the identifications of the contemplative mystics ; nor can the ecstasy of exhaustion produced by dancing, or the dreams due to drugs, be compared to the ecstasies of Buddhism or Christianity. It is not merely a question of degree. It is true that the same phenomena (granted that they are the same, though this is of rare occurrence), can be seen in the personalities of the normally constituted as well as in the mentally defective; but in normal cases the content has a universal value ; while in pathological cases the value is egotistical, and therefore doomed almost always to sterility.

Certainly in both cases we are dealing with uncommon personalities, eccentrics, or ' characters ' (at one time they were even spoken of as ' degenerates ') ; but mental disease, insanity, produces characters and eccentrics psychologically of a particular type and organically specific.

4. *Mysticism and Neurosis*

The most accredited authorities are content to refer the phenomena of mysticism to the neuroses rather than to insanity. This is another aspect of the controversy.

That the neuropath differs essentially from the dement is a point of view indispensable to a truly positive

psychiatry. The madman is socially valueless, but this is
not true of the neurotic. He may certainly give evidence
of a psychic rupture or imbalance equal to that of
insanity ; but it is not of such a nature as to constitute
a permanent deformation of behaviour. The psychic
personality possesses considerable resistance to temporary
extreme oscillations ; the cerebral damage is curable ;
the disturbances of character are at once recognized ;
morbid ideas can be corrected in the same way as are
mere errors of observation or judgment. The neurasthenic
may not only be the possessor of fine intellectual and
emotional capacity, but may also, in spite of his lacunæ,
be able to perform a series of actions directed towards
an end which is thoroughly justified by his own
intelligence. All this, therefore, excludes the arbitrary
supposition that the actions of neurasthenics and their
intellectual and affective products are the results of
isolated neuropathic symptoms.

There are some psychiatrists who would attribute
visions and voices to nervous exhaustion and neurosis.
There is, indeed, considerable truth in this idea. In
normal persons, however, once this exhaustion is past,
not only do the voices and visions cease, but those who
were subject to them are also able to criticize them
judiciously. When this does not occur, there are two
possibilities ; either the subject is a schizophrene or a
chronic paranoiac, and not a simple neuropath (asthenic) ;
or else he invests his visions, voices, dreams, and reveries
with faith, that is to say, with an interpretation supplied
by his religious belief. It is this added element which, as
has already been stated, characterizes the thoughts of the
mystic and gives them their value, not the mere fantastic
or sensory phenomenon.

It is, of course, indubitable that neuroses frequently

occur among exceptional personalities; and in 'exceptional' mystics and in the converted the neuroses may find an extraordinarily congenial field for their development.

In fact, according to Freud, the privation (*Versagung*) of the libido is the actual cause of nervous disorders. It is, however, also true—still according to Freud—that this privation may be tolerated without any adverse results. The ways of escape for the neurotic subject are various, once he has definitely shut off the broad road which Luther selected. The first form of escape consists in supporting privation with a certain nostalgia which lends a particular sadness to renunciation. The second is that of equivalents or substitutes, which are made possible by the great plasticity of the sexual instincts. The third is sublimation—either automatic or voluntary—with which we have already sufficiently dealt. From this it clearly results that the mystic's renunciation can easily be nostalgic, and that it can also be 'impure'; but that it need not of necessity descend to the level of pathological mysticism. Neither is the mystic fatally predestined to neurosis by reason of his renunciation.

But, it may be asked, are converts, like all mystics, when they appear to be exceptional personalities or types of character, to be deemed constitutionally predisposed or emotionally abnormal? Undoubtedly the neurotic constitution, as a stable condition, is to be found with noticeable frequency among the mystics and the more notable converts of our own times and of the past. The isolated symptoms of neurasthenia, hysteria, and depression are frequently present in them.

In particular there are certain psychiatrists who would consider the psychology of the converted generally as belonging to a variety of one of the two temperaments

distinguished by Kretschmer, more especially of the
'schizoid', or to the so-called constitutional cœnæsthopaths
described by Sollier, Deny, Camus, and Buscaino.   It is,
however, noteworthy that though the varieties of constitutional types (described by Viola) may throw some
light upon the peculiarities of the animal nervous system
and the endocrine glands, they offer no useful orientation
concerning the psychological characteristics.   In the
second place, the schizoid temperament which Kretschmer
bases upon the distant analogy of the symptomology
of schizophrenia, is too lacking in precise outlines to be
of use as a standard of reference.   We may, however,
observe in regard to the theory of cœnæsthopathy that the
physiology of cœnæsthesia is extremely poor in data,
and that the many hypotheses of psychopathology
which alienists have endeavoured to build upon it are
highly provisional and insecure.   In addition, the conception of cœnæsthopathy is so comprehensive that it
could be made to embrace all who in their psycho-
social life diverge from the human average.

The neurosis, or the cœnæsthopathy, of the converted
must, however, be examined more closely.   That the
affectivity of converts has something exceptional about
it is beyond question ; and that certain aspects of the
religious life are extra-logical because affective is also
certain.   On several occasions I have met in psychasthenics, even in the phase of acute depression, certain
experiences which deserve to be called mystic.   One
highly intelligent psychasthenic told me that she sometimes experiences a sort of ' change of position ' in respect
of her own ego or of her environment, so that she seems
to find herself in a different sphere, in which she feels
and sees inexpressible things.   This patient, who was
an unbeliever, asked me anxiously if what she felt was

not an experience of religious mysticism and whether it did not prove the existence of God and of the supernatural. In this case it is evident that the morbid element consisted not in the momentary ' depersonalization ', but in the anxiety—in the affective reaction. So too, among the schizophrenes we find the same experiences, but in these the morbidity consists only in the intellectual reaction (delirious ideas), and not in the actual experiences themselves, which are not intrinsically morbid, since there are experiences of this kind sufficiently often among normally intelligent persons, who are quite free from mental disease, and also in persons of artistic temperament.

A gulf, however, divides not merely morbid affectivity from delirium—in which the conceptual and rational systems are thrown into confusion, but also divides the affective excesses of certain mystics and converts from the emotionalism of hysterics and epileptoids, and again divides the exaltations of the mystics from the tachypraxia of the microsplanchnic hyperthyroidics or the ideo-affective dissociations of the schizothymes, and so forth.

The same thing may be said in regard to mental anguish. This darkening of the spirit is familiar to all religious souls ; but it is nevertheless true that the most poignant agony that can result from moral suffering or from remorse for sin or from non-morbid scruples, is not comparable with the anxiety of the melancholic, in whom the intellectual reactions differ so profoundly from those of both the normal and the neuropathic individual, or with the anguish of the psychasthenic such as that described by Janet, which is based on a ' sense of incompleteness '. Again, according to Blondel, the anguish suffered by the psychasthenic is undoubtedly an affective state, but it is a state *sui generis*, because it is fundamentally individualistic. It is 'pure affectivity', and as such differs from the affective experiences of individuals possessed of consciousness of the social type. It may at least be regarded, apart from Blondel's theory, as a persistent *état fort* or one recurring without logical motivation.

It seems useless to introduce fresh medical conceptions into the religious field to take the place of the old *neuropathic constitution*; but let it be thoroughly understood that constitution means the peculiarity of organic structure and temperament.[35]

The neuropathic diathesis (as well as, to a certain extent, the psychopathic) which is undoubtedly to be met with frequently among all exceptional persons and among the notable converts also, is nothing more or less than a form of individuality. To express this differently: it is an extreme variation of the personality—when it is not accompanied by a morbid process at some period of life. The neuropathic constitution must on no account be confused with insanity, even though the neuropath is less able than others to safeguard himself against insanity. To sum up: this constitutional tendency (neuro-psychopathic predisposition) like every other predisposition in medical science, is not pathological in respect of the characteristics which it actually presents, but rather in respect of the possibility of these characteristics embodying themselves in a morbid process when any favourable, but frequently unforeseen, opportunity occurs.

It should be added that while it is essential to distinguish between the constitution and the malady itself, it would also be useful to interpose between the two a further distinction. that of clinical orientation.

which I have already established for infantile neuro-psychiatry.[36]

By taking acrobatic leaps from possibility to probability—which should be based only on statistics—and from probability to actuality—which should be supported by direct observation—some psychiatrists have affirmed, in the name of science, the existence of insanity, epilepsy, hysteria, dysthymia, or schizothymia in all who have attracted public attention by reason of their exceptional thoughts or actions. Such alienists not only fall into evident logical fallacies, but into errors of technique in psychiatry, since the exceptional in behaviour becomes identified in their view with the neuro-psychopathic constitution—and what is still worse—this again is identified with insanity proper.

Such extremists are unconsciously returning to 'rational diagnosis'—which was known to the Alexandrian medical school and mentioned in the *Corpus Hippocrateum*—which dispensed with critical observations of phenomena and was based upon dialectic; or else they are turning towards the outworn theory of a 'morbid substance', which succeeded the doctrine of demoniacal possession of the Middle Ages and the belief in original sin, which had some supporters scarcely a century ago. According to this doctrine, once the morbid entity had entered the organism—as, for example, by heredity—it inevitably became the absolute master of the patient's personality; and it was revealed, now by combined somatic and psychic symptoms, now by psychic symptoms alone, thus demonstrating the hereditary fate of the so-called psychopathic constitution.

The same criticism should also be brought to bear upon the theory of the pathological degeneracy of genius.

It is not denied that one may find men of genius with somatic, psychic, or moral abnormalities; or that certain superior men have suffered from neurosis, psychosis, or true mental disease. Caravaggio, for instance, was a criminal; Sodoma was a homosexual; Schumann, Blake, Wiertz, Nietzsche, and Gemito were mentally affected. No one, however, has been able, up to the present, to isolate the 'specific' abnormality of the man of genius. This is only another way of saying that there are no serious arguments for regarding inventions, discoveries, or works of art as the 'direct products' of mental infirmity. At all events, it cannot be established that mental infirmity itself constitutes the specific, and therefore the only, stimulus of the highly intellectual temperament, and of the elaboration and the liberation of the subconscious, and of the production of works of genius. Fevers and chronic illnesses, like nervous affections, may sometimes provide the occasion for the expression of genius. An example of this is the case of the luetic Félicien Rops, with his tragic etchings directed against womankind. But it must be evident to everyone that content, stimulus, and capacity—or genius—are three entirely different conceptions.[37]

It is, in fact, so extremely difficult to demonstrate that a work of art is brought to perfection during the course of a psychosis or at the exact moment of the explosion of a psychic disturbance, that the audacious supporters of the pathological theory or theory of degeneration, like Moreau de Tours, Lombroso, and their disciples, were obliged to employ, in order to save their theory, a very curious method—that is, the paradox of 'equivalence', which involved a convenient but arbitrary extension of a clinical conception. According to this theory, the inventions of genius or artistic intuitions are to be regarded as the 'equivalents' of an epileptoid seizure or of a transient attack of insanity.[38] But the theory of equivalence is unsupported except by the sole and insufficient fact that both invention or intuition and the epileptic attack have a subconscious impetus. Everyone knows that this point of view is no longer held even by alienists, and in support of this statement I may mention my compatriots Morselli, Brugia, and Petrazzani, who are the authors of brilliant studies and monographs on the subject of degeneracy.

As a matter of fact, when one is considering either mad geniuses or insane saints, it is essential to admit one of two alternatives: either they were or are suffering intermittently from nervous or psychic disturbances, or else they are chronic paranoiacs or paranoids who yet are capable intermittently of intellectual or moral productions of considerable value. In both cases the identification of insanity with genius or saintliness is excluded.

No one would think of denying that there are religious souls tortured by true hallucinations or by other psychopathic symptoms, or who are actually alienated. But such coincidences, though of frequent occurrence, are capable of quite other explanations than the hypothesis of identity.

Neither empirical psychology nor psychiatry can agree to recognize that religious faith and devotion are 'specific' symptoms of disease or abnormality of the brain; or that mental disease constitutes the ordinary 'stimulus' to holiness or devoutness. The present-day technique of psychiatry is sufficiently advanced to recognize (in individuals present or absent) insane behaviour through its rapport with social activity. Insanity—

when it really exists—is manifest to the competent and disinterested psychiatrist.

The ' signs ' of insane behaviour are not merely the absurdity and inconstancy of purpose, incoherence of action, the pursuit of selfish aims, and so forth. The content of thought and action in insane subjects— in so far as this content consists of material derived from the subconscious—is almost passively accepted by the dement, and with only slight or summary control by the consciousness. This content he is unable to make his own, since he cannot elaborate it in accordance with intrinsic and extrinsic exigencies. A political, social, or religious reform, not inherently absurd, may reveal its insanity through its intemperance, which implies that it lacks an appropriate elaboration on the part of the subject. The work of the genius and the saint, it is true, has always a certain character of ' anticipation ' ; one might say that their specific social function consists in contributing interpretations of hidden needs in advance of current opinions. But with the lapse of years these interpretations meet with fulfilment, and this fulfilment may be foreseen by the superior minds of the period. There always comes a moment when a philosophical theory, a work of imagination, a mode of expression, or a reform, finds its appropriate reception and obtains from that age its true recognition.[39]

It may be concluded that modern psychopathology, having at present reached a maturity which it perhaps did not possess in previous decades, now has many scientific arguments to advance against certain theories and hypotheses of former times. The true mystics and the great converts, notwithstanding their neurotic qualities and certain incidental morbid symptoms, can be readily recognized and distinguished from mystics and converts who are insane or who are psycho-degenerates ; and this without having recourse to the usual loop-hole of 'value ', which is to some extent an extra-psychological argument. We may assume that the true mystics and converts are extreme variations in the field of the normal variation of human personality.

Finally, since we ourselves create our concepts and definitions, it should be agreed that mental alienation is a thing apart from mysticism, genius, and saintliness of life. In particular we would add that we ought not to speak of saintliness, or even of true religious conversion, in connection with cases in which the sublimation of the libido is inconstant or incomplete, unless we are speaking merely of the *phases of oscillation* in the conversional process.

CHAPTER VIII

SUMMARY AND CONCLUSION

THE PREDICTABILITY OF CONVERSION

IN this, our final chapter, we might be expected to present a recapitulation of the positions reached in this work, that is to say, a summary of the psychology of religious conversion. This, however, might not be a wise course, and might also, perhaps, occasion some misunderstanding. My intention is, instead, to illustrate psychologically, in accordance with modern scientific methods of religious psychology, one particular mode of conversion, almost specific to Catholicism—that form, in fact, which seems to me to exemplify what I have called *the typical conversional experience*.

In order to avoid the presumptuousness of too wide generalizations, and to relieve my exposition of those tiresome professorial airs which are quite out of place except in a text-book, I have conceived the notion of telling the story of an ' ideal convert ', who follows the course I have traced in the present work.

Fiction, however, does not seem the most suitable form in which to present what claims to be a scientific exposition of facts. I have accordingly drawn only on facts, and the account which follows represents a deliberate fusion of the actual stories of two separate converts— my Cases No. 2 and No. 3, both men of science, intellectual, cultured, and of a rationalistic bent. The biographical data in regard to place and time of both cases, and certain details in respect of testimony, different as might have been expected in the two subjects, would add nothing to the evidence. Moreover, the real essence of my work will be found in the explanatory psychological notes which I have interpolated in this history. I am indicating by the name of X my ' double ' convert.

X, in his infancy and boyhood, knew and practised the Catholic religion, without having—as is the case with every infant born and brought up in the traditional religious atmosphere—the slightest tendency to question the articles of faith taught him by his mother and by the catechism.

It must be borne in mind that a state of belief or faith is the ' normal ', or better the natural, state of infancy and childhood, just as it is in the infancy of the human race and in all the uncivilized peoples. In infancy, indeed, the representative and affective elements are not only welded together, but are fused together into a unitary ' psychic system ', owing to the paucity of the subject's experiences, and to his still feeble critical faculty.

Thus there were formed in X's mind not only the usual religious ' constellations ', products of imitation and of the memory of things read, heard, or seen, but true ideo-affective complexes charged with psycho-motor energy, that is, connected with the instincts of the species and with the most powerful personal interests.

These diminutive psychic solar systems of the mind exercise an attractive influence over other ideas, so that one may state that the whole of X's life, at a certain period in his childhood, was permeated by religiosity. His moral conduct was, in every respect, identical with that of boys of his age, educated or not according to

religious tradition.   His conduct alternated between
disciplined behaviour and rebellion ; his reading varied
from fantastic romances eagerly devoured, to obligatory
studies reluctantly pursued and intense preparations
for examinations successfully passed.

The tracks upon which childhood runs its course are
the same for all individuals : imagination, imitation,
amour-propre, and tendencies to freedom.

At twelve X felt the first torments of eroticism—true
escapes of repressed energy—which were easily calmed
down with the exterior aid of educational vigilance,
and the interior assistance of the fear of sin and the
duty of confessing it.   At the age of fourteen X was
at the height of the crisis of puberty—experiencing
interminable reveries, preoccupations with the success
of his school career, auto-eroticism, and, besides, an
already powerful passion for women, with vague
voluptuous dreams.   The crisis was displayed in a
notable deterioration both of character and conduct.
Doubts regarding religious matters were suggested
by his secondary studies, doubts which, little by little,
became stronger and led eventually to complete religious
indifference.

In this fashion the infantile religious complexes came
to be gradually removed, little by little, from the level
of conscious actuality, and sank deep into the obscurity
of the subconscious, where their reduced power was
insufficient to raise them to the level of consciousness.
The now established religious indifference naturally
inhibited all outbursts of repentance.

Throughout his adolescence X was dominated by
sensual love.   The two psychic systems—erotic and
cultural—are always at the fore-front of conscious
activity in adolescence.   The old tendencies and the habits

of faith are inhibited ; and in consequence, the repressed complexes of childhood and youth sink deeper and deeper into the subconscious.

In fact the fever for knowledge and the fever of his sexual desires and, in a lesser degree, interest in his material prospects, preoccupied almost the entire daily existence of young X between his fifteenth and his eighteenth years.

No notable changes occurred in the years following. This would imply that the psychic energy had succeeded in attaining a ' systemization ', which apparently had become definitive. X, in fact, throughout the period between his twenty-second and thirtieth years, was a radical in politics and a free-thinker in philosophy ; and, as he was a student of the natural sciences, he was also a fanatical evolutionist. Habit and convention slowly crystallized the youthful convictions so intensely experienced in regard to the sciences, art, politics, and his professional activity. Thus the secondary psychic systemization, which had superseded the primary systemization of infancy and adolescence, became firmly consolidated.

In spite of good fortune, however, X's life had its thorns. On various occasions domestic misfortune, illness, isolation, and certain shattered illusions of love turned his mind towards unwonted reflections.

This indicated a lowering of tension in the psychic systems formed in youth, that is, the second systemization. And then, between X's thirtieth and fortieth years, a certain causeless restlessness appeared. This we may interpret as a deviation of energy, due to an alteration in the regime of the complexes.

Mutations of the character are conscious processes. They are rationalized, and the reason supplies excellent, but not invariably consistent, justifications. In spite of new and studiously sought-for pleasures, and in spite of providential changes in his circumstances, this profound restlessness still remained in X's soul. He sought relief in pleasure, in philosophy, and in sociology, and finally he had recourse to theosophy. This constitutes what X himself terms his ' philosophic period '.

In reality it was an unconscious deviation of energy into new channels, and the second systemization was suffering in consequence.

There followed alterations in X's habits, indulgence of his amour-propre, roseate hopes, days of calm, illusions, fresh internal conflicts, and still uneasinesses of every sort. Nevertheless he ultimately succeeded in feeling, at this period, master of his own inner mental situation. During the three or four years before he reached the age of forty he kept himself well under control. He appeared to have succeeded in obtaining that complete ' unification ' of the psychic personality to which he had aspired for so many years. The philosophic period had not brought him either good fortune or peace, but his work, his family life, and the distractions of love had cured him of his uneasiness.

Here we discover a fresh systemization, the third, corresponding to the fullness of his psychic development. Henceforth, X's life flowed on in perfect tranquillity, almost happily. This new systemization continued unabated for several years.

Somewhere between the ages of forty and forty-two, and by a pure coincidence, X was present at some religious ceremony. It made a rather pleasant impression on him. A few days later he chanced to be reading a novel (Sienkiewicz's *Without Dogma*, in the case of one of my two subjects). He was much impressed. A few weeks later he chanced to meet the old confessor of his school days, an encounter which seemed to him strange, but which was not so in reality. This provoked in him a certain state of ' opening of the mind ', as if suddenly he understood much that hitherto had been incomprehensible. What he had been learning in theosophy he was now able to complete. He experienced an extraordinary sensation, as if all at once he felt the hollowness of many things which he had held to be unimpugnable truths. After this he had transient perceptions of meanings, intuitions, and psychic depression. These, however, proved only momentary and produced no permanent alterations either in the character or habits of the fortunate professional man. But one day in his forty-first year clearly defined childhood memories of a religious nature appeared in X's consciousness.

Here the complex deeply immersed in the subconscious mind had momentarily risen *en bloc* to consciousness, bringing up with it its affective component—the state of faith—with unimpaired vivacity and force.

From this moment onwards his uneasiness increased. At intervals of reflection he would frankly put to himself the question of a ' return ' to his old faith. He then began reading Christian apologetics.

It is evident that at this period the levels of his cultural and sexual complexes must have been slowly sinking, and that it was this fact which facilitated the emergence, with revivified energy, of the old infantile complexes.

On special occasions X experienced for some moments all the ingenuous childlike state of faith, accompanied by an interior commotion, followed by a sense of profound calm. One such mystical experience happened to him in the country, in silence and solitude, with the panorama of nature before his eyes. This strange sensation, almost of happiness, made him desire the repetition of the experience. Finally he determined to make an effort to conquer it.

What did such a conquest imply? Nothing other than the transformation of memories of beliefs and desires into actual beliefs and desires, that is, a fulfilment of desires. X steadily advanced towards a change, and this procedure—as the reader should note—was fully conscious.

Now it was exactly at this period that X's true struggles began. This shaking off of old mental habits, and the forming of new ones is always accompanied by profound disturbances. His reason balked; his customs protested; the habits of a lifetime were a definite obstruction to any return towards the religion of his childhood.

One morning in his forty-second year, as he was reading, he was once more forcibly confronted by the 'infantile religious complex', an automatic appearance due to the vigour of the complex. On the occasion of this encounter the complex was accepted by the fully conscious mind. It was a categorical affirmation, accompanied by a sense of victory and of liberation—almost of frenzy. After a few hours, however, the 'yes' was withdrawn. The conflicting considerations of his environment, of his habits, rose within X. His mode of life could not adapt itself, and, in consequence, his religious convictions suddenly became feebler. All the arguments of science and of history then became effective obstacles. The uselessness of religion, the illogicality of faith, were strongly evident.

After a few months, however, these objections were

once more overcome; the motives for belief were once more accepted. But this was not conversion; it was merely the confirming of a ' pre-mutation '.

The affective component of an emergent infantile complex requires reinforcement, which may be slow in arriving, or very often never comes at all, as in cases of pseudo-conversion or pre-conversion. Or this re-energizing may occur in old age, or during a serious illness, at which times the suggestions and emotions of fear become more powerful.

Then one day X had a new and crushing disillusion in love, losing the sweetheart of many years. Shortly after his pride also suffered a blow. He then experienced a true inward mutation; that is to say, his tastes, his desires, his mode of life, all became altered. But this was obviously not a sudden conversion.

At this point a displacement of psychic energy became apparent, implying a transference of affective energy to a more ideal object. And this object, now perfectly ' clear to consciousness ' was already waiting. The act of transference, however, as is most natural, was automatic—and therefore unconscious—since the subject himself had not observed the passage of energy, but only became conscious that his energy had already been transferred.

As time went on, X realized more clearly the actuality of the transference, going over the process of his mutation in memory. Now he recognized and interpreted his conversion; and like all converts, he attributed it to ' grace ', not because he felt his own *extraneousness* to the fact of his mutation—a phenomenon admitted by the American psychologists—but because he felt that he had been helped by Providence to turn his steps towards a new objective, so much worthier than the old.

(This distinction was categorically made to me by both my converted subjects during the course of interrogation, or, as it is called, ' induced introspection '.)

The sublimation is evident. But in X even this phase of the conversional process was unconscious. When he recognized that his sentiments of veneration, of discipline, and of love had been directed toward a higher aim, he had the sense of having been " helped by ' grace ' " in his difficult ascent.

It is true that the affective energy had already been transferred and sublimated by the time that X was able to recognize himself as changed; but he had himself prepared for the process of sublimation by his efforts and sacrifice, and he now maintained his sublimation in his full consciousness, and with the will at full tension, while he resisted the continual and sometimes powerful impulses towards his former state. And this implies an incessant renewal of his sublimation, occurring in full consciousness. X, indeed, confessed that he had suffered and rejoiced much during this period of trial.

The oscillation between suffering and rejoicing lasts until the sublimation has become habitual. This may happen late or may never occur at all.

Religious conversion is in reality a complex and gradual psychic process in which the whole personality undergoes a complete mutation. It is prepared by individual conditions over a long period, analogous to the ' pre-mutations ' of biology; a preparation which only in very exceptional cases remains wholly unknown to the subject himself. The process consists in a re-arrangement of the ideo-affective-motor complexes of the individual, more or less definitely induced by exterior causes, sometimes in the form of crises. This recasting is only a fresh systemization of the affective energy—or of the individual *pathos*. It is displayed in the sphere of morals by a process of sublimation and elevation of pride, of love, and of the emotional life in general. It is, therefore, a new economy of love.

The process of conversion, like all biological mutations, presents a longer or shorter period of adjustment or adaptation, ' the period of oscillation ' But if the conversion is genuine, it invariably ends in a new equipoise of thought and life.

It would be erroneous to reduce the entire process to an automatism. Both history and experience teach that true conversion consists in the subject's awareness— though it may not be continuous—of his mutation and of its aim. He must accept the mutation itself more or less completely and with his will, either rapidly or after a long period of painful conflict and of sacrifice. His conversion, whether it arrives by crises or by gradual steps, must be lived, the subject finding in it his mental stability, and the reason and the joy of existence.

In X, habitual sublimation had evidently not yet appeared. Occasionally he experienced days of discomfort and of ' aridity '. However, by the sixth decade of his life, his conversion had become sufficiently established and his life was serene. The signs that X had accomplished a profound affective mutation are numerous. They consist in fresh interpretations of reality in place of the old explanations of his philosophic days ; in a sense of happiness, or at least of peace ; in a more or less vivid ' sense of presence ' ; and, further, in a veneration and tenderness towards God, the Madonna, and the Church.

When crises of depression occur, accompanied by unhappiness and by the usual doubts, they do not suffice to destroy the harmony of our convert's existence.

Even now, however, he does not like to be confronted by the objections of logic, history, or science. He avoids certain intellectual arguments because he desires to believe and is determined to remain a Catholic in spite of everything.

X has certainly changed some of his former daily habits, although he still continues the regular practice of his profession. The woman who is his companion has assumed a particular value for him; his senses are appeased, while his mind is chaste. In this case we find a true sublimation of love, in love.

There are two new habits which have developed in our convert's life since his conversion: *prayer* and *charity*. The latter has assumed a character entirely different from the almsgiving of his earlier life. The poor not only arouse his sense of compassion, but he loves them and envies their freedom, since they will have nothing to regret leaving when they die. (This confession was made to me, on inquiry, by both converts.) At times X feels an impulse to become like the poor, at all events in certain aspects. Here we find in X a clear initiation of 'affective identification', however momentary. An identification of this kind, which is 'endopathic', may become conscious and volitional, in other words, active, 'willed', and almost a vent for tenderness. But this experience is not found among X's confessions.

In prayer our convert finds great repose, and he has the sensation of Christ and the Virgin near him; a clear 'sense of presence'.

To-day, after a lapse of some fifteen years since his mutation, X is tranquil and calm, although attached to life, to his family, and to his studies. In the lives of both of the converts whose experiences I have just described there is no appearance of serious nervous disturbances or of any psychopathic crises.

Before concluding, I must respond to a demand which will naturally be raised by my readers. If my analysis is to be regarded as scientific, it must supply some criteria for predicting the occurrence of conversion in individuals who come under our observation. *Savoir pour prevoir, et prevoir pour pourvoir*: in that motto is included all science with all its ends.

The theologian would, of course, at once take exception to this demand, since according to his doctrine a transcendental and therefore unpredictable factor takes part in every conversion, that is, ' grace '. But even the theologian may ask some information of the psychologist. Dante says :

> . . . *sie certo*
> *che ricever la grazia è meritorio*
> *secondo che l'affetto l'è aperto.*
>
> (*Paradiso*, XXIX, 64–66.) *

' *L'apertura dell' affetto* ', 'the opening of the desire ', is essentially a psychological phenomenon which can be foreseen. Therefore one cannot but refer to the individual biological and psychological phenomena which intervene in the process of conversion.

The physiological conditions of the subjects concerning whom we wish to make a prediction can enlighten us very little, not because of intrinsic reasons, but because of our ignorance of the field. Importance has been assigned both to the age of the subject and to the conditions and functioning of his internal secretions, but such data are too general, even when they are not altogether

---

* " Be certain that to receive grace is meritorious, in proportion as the desire is laid open to it."

equivocal. The modern doctrine of 'constitutions' also fails to supply us with any positive data; for instance, it is valuable to draw the clinical picture of constitutional hyperthyroidism or hypogenitalism, but in addition to the humours there are always the nervous system and the cerebral cortex which determine the destiny of the libido. Kretschmer lays stress on the well-known fact of dissociation between genitalism and psychic sexuality, which is a normal phenomenon at puberty, but which is prolonged in subjects of the astheno-schizothymic temperament because of the under-development of the genital glands and other hormonic anomalies (according to Pende's investigations) or more frequently because of hyperthyroidism. Observation of the astheno-schizothymic temperament—if such a temperament actually does exist—cannot, however, give us any data specific enough to be of service in making predictions. A state of vital hypotonia, when verified, may be considered a favourable condition, but only for the *initiation* of the conversional process. In any event, vital hypotonia is of importance for us only in so far as it is a concomitant of a psychic condition. For hypovitality is translated into consciousness as suffering; and suffering evokes a desire for its opposite, since none long for felicity and peace as do those who suffer and struggle. It is the psychic conditions of the individual, therefore, which should attract the attention of the psychologist who attempts prognostication.

Since the act of volition, which is the most essential factor in conversion, is the least easily foreseen of human activities, our attempt at prognostication may seem rash. But every volition must have a substance which it kindles. The practical spirit of men, as Benedetto

Croce says, operates upon an 'historical situation', without which there could be no volition. One may admit as freely as one will Varisco's theory of 'auto-determination' before a multiplicity of motives, and choice between a plurality of excitants, and election among countless and diverse attractions—nevertheless, we must still discover the material on which volition is to work. Now the individual historic situation, albeit variable, may be *foreseen*, because it is, at bottom, an actuality and can therefore be *seen* by those who are capable of seeing it. The question as to the possibility of prediction is affirmatively answered not only by realists, since science is the exact knowledge of causes, but also by the idealists, since for them the principle of causality corresponds to the unity of the spirit with itself.

However, it is certain that psychological prediction is relative. It is limited by the presence of voluntary action and of profound individual historical situations, which are necessarily invisible, as well as by interference coming from fields of experience which are totally different and thus contingent and unpredictable. In spite of this limitation, however, the actual and visible signs of the conversional process may be noted. We should never forget that conversion, as we regard it, is a *normal* phenomenon, an individual psychic evolution both theoretically and practically distinct from any morbid process. And it is on this account that conversion, though to a limited extent, can be both systematized and predicted.

Great precision and great completeness are not to be expected in this exposition. It is not intended to do more at the present time than offer the psychologist a general orientation. The variations, the exceptions, the atypical cases, and the whole series of unforeseen factors can be easily added by the reader. Those psychic situations favourable for the occurence of religious conversion of an individual may be considered to be the following :—

First—The presence of general religious tendencies or ' religiosity ', deriving either from heredity, from the family, or from impressions in the infancy or childhood of the individual, from that age, in fact, when the formation of ' psychic systems ' is most active, strong, and free, owing to the greater plasticity of the psyche and of the brain, and to the immaturity of the will. Infancy and childhood are the ages during which the material of future adult volitions is prepared.

No one can fail to recognize the two most potent factors of religious mutations throughout life—by which I mean the inborn disposition of the subject, and the education received during the earliest years. Even religiosity is an hereditary echo. The question of psychological heredity is much discussed, but though interpretations vary, the phenomenon is undeniable. The results of the researches of the Dutchmen, Heymans and Wiersma, summarized by Bühler, on the heredity of psychic qualities, have demonstrated that such qualities are inherited in 97·6 per cent of the cases. The influence of environment, as seen in early education, has never been questioned. It can be broadly assumed that the harvest in after life corresponds with the seed sown during early years by the family and the school. Here the reader should recall the case of Ernest Renan. He has himself told us of the influence of his mixed heredity, part Breton, part Gascon, on his variable temperament—which was at once reflective and mystic, thoughtless and sceptical. Renan has faithfully placed on record the clearest evidence of the influence of heredity and education, first on his mysticism and later on his incredulity.

Second—An habitual tendency of the intellect towards absolute convictions, whether affirmative or negative, in respect of philosophy, theology, politics, etc. This mental make-up will be easily understood if it is described as the antithesis of the critical attitude.

Third—A tendency of the individual spontaneously to fix the attention beyond and above the realities of the senses. This tendency is analogous to the physical accommodation of the eye to infinity, in other words, its focussing upon far distant objects—so analogous in fact, that in the state of reverie the ocular axes actually tend to become parallel (dreamy-eyed). This tendency is accompanied by an attitude of mind, that of abstraction from the immediate surroundings and of contemplation of more profound objects and aims, which are by nature obscure. This mental tendency leads on one hand to a sense of the mysterious, and on the other to a spirit of renunciation of immediate material enjoyment in order to obtain a felicity of a more lasting and universal character.

Such a condition is found in its most striking form in persons of the so-called artistic temperament, and in the normal mystics. It is certain that there are people who seem to lend their ears to the distant voices of the past (subconscious) while other people seem deaf to them, intent and fixed only upon the immediate realities.

Fourth—A richness of affective potential, which can be ascertained in the conscious sphere of practical life or in the subconscious, by analysis of the behaviour and attitude of the subject, or by the Freudian technique of psycho-analysis.[1] In the Freudian phraseology, such affective potential is the amount of energy (*Libidobetrag*) which the subject can hold in suspension.

The so-called warm temperament (and by temperament is meant not a mere assemblage of habits and attitudes, as so many affirm, but all this, plus the *pathos*), which is always associated with a vivid imagination, is always an indication of such high potential. Religious history records two great converts—St. Paul and St. Augustine—in whom passion was equal to genius.

Modern medical science has been searching for the organic and nervous correlations of this temperament. We may say—taking into account what little we do know in this connection, or rather what we postulate— that the endocrine formula most favourable to radical mutations in life and thought is the hyperthyroid-hyperpituitary–hypergenital–hypo-adrenal. The reader must pardon this rapid excursion into such uncertain territory.

It is of greater interest to observe that those who have an exuberant affective life are more prone than others to rapid alterations of mood and emotion. This, it seems to me, may explain why dysthymia and more especially cyclothymia appear with such frequency among converts and those who are verging towards conversion. The mere tendency to ' fickleness of mind ', however, must not be taken as an indication of mental illness.

Fifth—The existence of displacements or temporary transferences, either slow or violent, of the affective force, to groups of representations or particular ideas whose content recalls the ethico-religious ' psychic systems '. In short, the tendency of the individual to transfer his chief interests to questions of origin, purpose, destiny, and so forth.

A richness of affective potential, in association with a facility for its displacement and transference, is characteristic of all enthusiasts and fanatics. What Renan wrote of St. Paul therefore contains no disparagement : " *Paul était prés d'aimer ce qu'il haïssait.*"

Sixth—The recurrence of painful experiences ; to these we must assign more importance as a criterion of predicting the occurrence of conversion when their external reactions are deeper and less visible ; which leads one to believe that these experiences are causing an accumulation (repression) of affective energy rather than a release or dissipation of it.

The presence of these ' situations ' in an individual may make for the probability of his religious conversion, that is to say, powerful volitional processes will probably take possession of such material and kindle it as soon as the great passions of sensuality and pride have been subdued, and the reason has acquiesced and accepted the common motives for belief in God and in the individual values beyond physical existence.

The probability is much greater when one is dealing with multitudes, masses of individuals. This is easily understood when we reflect that the volitional acts of the mass are incomplete ; that we are here dealing with ' mere willing ', as various psychologists, including Wundt, have expressed it, and not with complete volitions. On this probability is based the propaganda for religious conversion ; and as statistics demonstrate, such propaganda throughout the ages has produced fixed and secure results whenever the conditions remain unaltered.[2]

NOTES AND BIBLIOGRAPHY

CHAPTER I

[1] E. Claparède, VI International Congress of Psychology, Geneva, 1909; *Rapports et Communications* (Geneva, 1910). This contains a full report of the discussion on religious psychology.

[2] The term *psychologie religieuse* was due to the late Professor Th. Flournoy, of Geneva, who took part in the discussions with enthusiasm. This distinguished authority had already maintained for some years (see *Archives de Psychologie*, Geneva, 1903), that psychology should exclude the consideration of the transcendental objects of religion. Th. Ribot, also, maintained that psychology may analyze, but has no competence to discuss, the objective value of religious emotions. Hence it would seem that the limits of psychological research in religious phenomena are defined by a sufficient consensus of opinion. Those who philosophize whenever mention is made of religious facts are not psychologists, but philosophers, of either the positivist or the spiritualist school. Naturally many psychologists have been concerned with such subjects as faith, holiness, religious feeling, conversion, and so forth. Luigi Valli deals with the subject in a brief but capable monograph, *Il fondamento psicologico della religione* (Rome, 1904); in which the author accepts, for the most part, the views of Wundt. Others, both before and after Flournoy, have supported the view which we may call the agnostic theory of religious psychology. Read, for example, Renda's article " La teoria psicologica dei valori " in *Bilychnis*, October and November, 1920. This writer contends that psychology does not discuss the ' value ' of the content of our states of consciousness. A book by T. K. Oesterreich may be recommended in which these various questions are treated with method and clearness : *Einführung in die Religionspsychologie* (Berlin, 1917). Furthermore, a good bibliographical orientation upon religious psychology is to be found in the " Revue et bibliographie générale de psychologie religieuse ", in the *Archives de psychologie* (Geneva, February, 1914) ; it is a comprehensive survey.

For the method of religious psychology, in addition to the writings of Flournoy, I may indicate the *Études d'histoire et de psychologie du mysticisme*, by Henri Delacroix (Paris, 1908). The scientific method is followed by A. Gemelli, in his *L'origine sub-cosciente dei fatti mistici*, 3rd edition, with bibliographical appendix (Florence). This author belongs to the scientific school, but he includes a certain amount of critical and polemical matter ; cf. Chap. IV, p. 51 et seq.

[3] The words of Father Pacheu will be found in the Report of the Congress of Geneva, op. cit.

[4] Cf. the review *Les Études*, Paris, 1910.

[5] G. Truc, " Grâce et foi " in the *Revue philosophique*, July, 1914. This author has also published : *La Grâce, Essai de psychologie religieuse, Grâce et foi, L'État de grâce, Les états mystiques négatifs, La sainteté*. One vol. (Paris, 1920).

[6] The note referred to occurs in Höffding's *Philosophy of Religion* (London, 1906), cf. *Filosofia della Religione* (Turin, 1909).

[7] God is not an object of psychology, as some maintain. Leuba well says that if God were to be revealed to the interior consciousness it would be an empiric God. Read Xavier Moisant : *Dieu: l'expérience en métaphysique* (Paris, 1907), a most interesting book for those desiring to become oriented in the application of the scientific method in theodicy and apologetics.

[8] J. H. Leuba, " Les tendences fondamentales des mystiques chrétiens," in the *Revue philosophique*, July and August, 1902.

[9] The encyclical letter of Pope Pius X, dated 8th September, 1907, on the subject of Modernist doctrines is known to all. The reader of Italian may study it, preceded by a succinct study of Modernism, in Giuseppe Prezzolini's *Cos'è il modernismo?* (Milan, 1908).

[10] This is to be found in the Report of the Congress of Geneva, op. cit., and in the pages of the *Archives de psychologie*. To be still further oriented cf. Théodore Flournoy's *Psychologie religieuse*.

[11] On the subject of contemporary psychology and its limits, the reader may consult any of the following studies by myself : " Psicologia sperimentale ", " Di alcune tendenze della psicologia contemporanea ", " Il metodo nella psicologia criminale e giudiziaria ", all of which appeared in *Contributi psicologici del laboratorio di psicologia sperimentale di Roma* (vol. iii, 1914-17) ; also " G. Wundt e la psicologia sperimentale ", in the same publication (vol. iv, 1922).

I would refer the over-optimistic scientist who believes that the renunciation of Psychologism for Agnosticism is a sympton of weakness in modern psychology, to the words of the celebrated French physiologist, Charles Richet : "*Il faut être solidement persuadé que la science d'aujourd'hui pour vraie qu'elle soit, est terriblement incomplète.*"

[12] The recent monograph of Georg Runtze contains a maximum of philosophy and a minimum of psychology :

" Psychologie der Religion " in Kafka's *Handbuch der vergleichenden Psychologie*, vol. ii (Munich, 1922), with an excellent bibliography.

[13] Benedetto Croce, *Cultura e vita morale—Intermezzi polemici* (Bari, 1914), p. 61.

[14] Cf. Giovanni Gentile, *Il Modernismo e i rapporti tra religione e filosofia* (Bari, 1921). The idealist says : when I reason, I mould the facts according to my thoughts in order to make them true ; facts cannot be truth unless I possess, more or less consciously, the criterion of truth ; therefore, categorical thought dominates everything. But this philosophy contains a whole theory of religion which transcends our scope. If we were only concerned to know how the convert arrives at the conviction of transcendency, and what power he gains from it, that would be within our scope ; but since the existence of external reality—the non-ego—is a postulate (and not a dogma) of empirical psychology, it becomes clear that such investigations surpass the limitations of psychology itself. This, however, does not mean that science may not legitimately advance explanatory hypotheses. Quite otherwise ; in fact, anthropologists, sociologists, philosophers, both ancient and modern, as well as psychopathologists, have advanced many and diverse hypotheses. For instance, the need of man completely to overcome fear, or to objectivate and give value to his most secret aspirations ; the animistic or magic tendency ; the existence of a special religious emotion ; the sense of the presence of the Absolute ; the sense of the infinite ; impotence of the will ; and the neuroses. These are a few of the theories. All of these, as against the theories of immanence or of transcendentalism, have this advantage : that they at least are hypotheses which start from facts, in other words, they arrive at their conclusions by induction ; the others, on the contrary, are doctrines, that is, unarguable certainties and therefore ultra-empirical.

[15] At the Geneva Congress of 1909 Bertrand declared that the psychology of religion should employ the Method of Residues of John Stuart Mill, according to which it was to be established that whatever remained of a religious phenomenon, which was not explicable by natural causes—either psychological, physiological, or historical—should be considered as caused by God. The contrary theory was propounded by Höffding, who argued that the residuum is the unknown. This, of course, is perfectly well understood by the psychologist.

[16] Th. Mainage, *La Psychologie de la Conversion*, 3rd edition (Paris, 1919), contains a good bibliography. This author is an ardent supporter of the doctrine of ' grace ' (*Educateur invisible*), though he claims to be concerned with the psychology, and not

with the theology, of conversion. Certain Catholics have found much to complain of in the methods adopted by Father Mainage. With these reservations, this book, like all the rest of the writings of Mainage, is a most interesting discussion of conversion. I have made use of it to a great extent in the present work.

[17] G. Berguer has dealt on several occasions with the psychology of religion, and also with psycho-analysis in connection with Jesus. The same author has published the (already cited) " Revue et bibliographie générale de psychologie religieuse " in the *Archives de Psychologie*. Father Mainage alludes to Berguer in the foreword of his *Psychologie de la Conversion*, op. cit.

[18] Renda, *La validità della Religione* (Città di Castello, 1921).

[19] Edwin Diller Starbuck, who is one of the chief American authorities on the subject, has written various contributions to the subject of religion, several of which will be quoted later on. Meanwhile, I would remind the reader of his " Contributions to the Psychology of Religion " in the *American Journal of Psychology*, ix, 1897. The author's ideas are expounded in his book *The Psychology of Religion : An Empirical Study of the Growth of Religious Consciousness* (preface by William James, 1899). This book has been translated into German (Leipzig, 1909), and Starbuck's work has been much quoted and commented on by German writers, particularly by Ernst Meumann in his *Vorlesungen zur Einführung in die experim. Pädagogik u. ihre psychol. Grundlagen* (Leipzig, 1911), vol. i, p. 614 et seq.

[20] William James's *Varieties of Religious Experience* has been translated into Italian by G. C. Ferrari and Calderoni (Turin, 1904). It consists of a splendid series of lectures, and is an indispensable preliminary to the study of the psychology of religion. It is to be recommended most strongly, and particularly Lecture I, on Religion and Nervous Pathology, Lecture VIII, on Cases of Counter-Conversion, and Lecture IX, on Conversion.

[21] Dr. Binet-Sanglé, *La folie de Jésus* (2nd edition, Paris, vol. i, 1909, vol. ii, 1910). The first volume treats of the heredity, the constitution, and the physiology of Jesus Christ. In the second volume His learning, ideas, delusions, and hallucinations are dealt with. This book, which has been called impious, has no scientific, historical, medical, or psychological value.

[22] Stanley Hall, *Jesus the Christ in the Light of Psychology* (New York, 1917, London, 1923, 2 vols.). The author considers the figure of Jesus as the spirit of his race. He says in effect : Jesus is the greatest projection of the popular soul (the Folk-soul) that has ever occurred. The book deals with every aspect of Jesus, but particularly with the psychological and racial origins of the beliefs about the personality of Christ. The work is a psychological interpretation of the personality of Christ,

especially in the light of genetic and social psychology, and of the Freudian doctrine.

[23] Psycho-analysis in the Freudian sense is too well-known through German, English, and Italian publications to need separate mention. Sigmund Freud's own published writings on the subject are already very voluminous. A good Freudian bibliography is to be found in Smith Ely Jelliffe's work, *The Technique of Psycho-analysis* (New York and Washington, 1920), of which we shall have occasion to make further mention. A more recent Freudian bibliography is given in *Sigmund Freud, his Personality, his Teaching, and his School*, by Fritz Wittels (London, 1924). If the non-medical reader (of Italian) cares to orient himself further on this branch of psychology, he can do so easily by consulting the articles of Dr. Assagioli appearing in the review *Psiche* (Florence) ; or the more technical works of Levi-Bianchini, whose bibliography is given in the *Archivo Generale di Neurologia, Psichiatria e Psicoanalisi* (Nocera Inferiore and Naples). Bianchini's " La dinamica dei psichismi secondo la psicoanalisi ", communicated to the Seventh International Congress of Psycho-Analysis, held in Berlin in September, 1922, is published with a bibliography, in the *Arch. Gen. di Neur. Psichiatr. e Psicoanal.* (Naples, 1922).

[24] F. Morel, *Essai sur l'introversion mystique, étude psychologique du pseudo Denys l'areopagite et de quelques autres cas de mysticisme* (Geneva, 1918), p. 338. The author mentions St. Bernard of Clairvaux, Bl. Henry Suzo, Madame Guyon, the pseudo Dionysius, and others.

See also the critique of the book by Th. Reik in his synthetic review in the *Bericht über die Fortschritte der Psychoanalyse in den Jahren 1914–19* (Vienna, Leipzig, Zurich, 1921), p. 229.

In the same *Bericht* it appears, according to Jung, that the introversion of the libido occurs when the world of fantasy is overloaded by *Libidoquantitäten*, and is the preliminary step (*Vorstufe*) to the formation of mystical symptoms. The libido in these cases is cut off from reality, and the subject's thoughts are occupied exclusively with such fantasies as the ego will tolerate on account of their *Harmlosigkeit*, or innocuousness. See p. 95 of the *Bericht*.

[25] Otto Rank and H. Sachs, *Die Bedeutung der Psychoanalyse für die Geisteswissenschaften* (Wiesbaden, 1913) ; O. Rank, *Das Inzestmotiv in Dichtung und Sage* (Leipzig and Vienna, 1912) ; and especially Reik, *Probleme der Religionspsychologie* (Leipzig, 1919). This last book, with a preface by Sigmund Freud, has as its motto a quotation from St. Paul's Epistle to the Romans xi, 18 : " Boast not against the branches. But if thou boast, thou bearest not the root, but the root thee."

According to Freud's preface to Reik's work, the ego is not capable of extirpating or of annulling the spiritual forces opposed to its own cultural ideas, but which it has removed as contrary to, or disintegrating to, its unity. The ego, therefore, leaves such conceptions in the primitive level and proceeds to protect itself against their assaults by energetic efforts of defence and offence. Or else it adopts the other expedient of endeavouring to accommodate itself to them through satisfactory surrogates. Directly these forces are displaced in a manner unfavourable to the ego, dreams or psycho-neuroses are the result.

The psycho-analysts in their study of ethnographic and pre-historical material, have interpreted religious origins, from totemism onwards, as possessing one common factor : that God the Father had at one time walked in person upon the earth, and as chief of a tribe of primitive men abused his powers of domination, so that his sons united to kill him ; and that, moreover, as the effect of this liberating crime, and as a compensatory expiation of it, there arose the first social ties, the first moral and social restrictions, and totemism, the most ancient form of religion. And so, too, all the religions that have subsequently arisen are filled with the same content ; and while they endeavour to eliminate all traces of this crime, or to expiate it, substituting other situations for the fight between father and sons, still they cannot avoid reiterating the elimination of the father. In mythology also we find the reverberations of this old memory, which throws a gigantic shadow over the development of the human race. Cf. Sigmund Freud, *Totem und Tabu* (Vienna, 1913). English translation by A. A. Brill, *Totem and Taboo, Resemblances Between the Psychic Lives of Savages and Neurotics* (New York and London, 1918, 1919).

In his first volume Reik bases his theories upon this hypothesis in order to interpret the problems of religious psychology. As point of departure he takes certain details of religious life found at the present day, and of religions among primitive races, archaic peoples, and neuropaths, and proceeds to explain them. The neurotic is the survival of archaic and primitive culture and experience. The hysteric is a poet, in that his own imaginings embody themselves dramatically, regardless of the understanding of other people. Thus the inhibitions and the ceremonials of the compulsive psycho-asthenics show that they have created their own private religion. So, too, the ideas of the paranoiacs display an external resemblance and an inward kinship to the systems of the philosophers. These patients therefore seek for the solution of their conflicts in precisely the same fashion as do the artists and the philosophers (through poetry, religion, or philosophy), but the latter resolve them in accordance with the needs of society. According to the statements of Reik in the Introduction to the book just quoted, psycho-analytical researches investigate, but do not exhaust, religion. Its preoccupation is with the subconscious side of religion. It refers to the ceremonial practices, which are of importance as the small acts of a patient are of significance in the course of an illness. The two factors, however, of chief importance in the moulding of the destiny of any race are *Anlage* or predisposition, and *Erleben* or experience. There can be no doubt that the ante-natal experiences are a most important influence on life.

[26] The study of religion can be made, according to Durkheim, only by observation of its exterior effects upon the life of the community. The same opinion is held by Wundt. But Leuba maintains that the comprehension of religion requires that its results should be explained in terms of consciousness. Religion should also be studied by the psychological method, i.e. through introspection. To this Durkheim objects that the social consciousness is entirely different from that of the individual, just as bronze is entirely different from the tin, copper, and lead of which it is composed. The human elements of society, however, are not physical or chemical substances, and the mentality of groups is conformable to laws quite different from the laws which govern the individual ; but if the collective group has a group-consciousness, a group-mentality, may not that be psychologically studied ? The studies of the sociologists are of great importance, and especially in regard to the development of the religious sentiment, as well as the relationship of the positive religions with social development. Cf. Emil Durkheim, *Les formes élémentaries de la vie religieuse. Le système totémique en Australie* (Paris, 1912) ; *Les règles de la méthode sociologique* (Paris, 1910).

See also G. W. Cooke, *The Social Evolution of Religion* (Boston, 1920), vol. iii, p. 416. Cooke studies the development of religion in its relation to social development in the Spencerian sense.

Richard Thurnwald, " Psychologie des primitiven Menschen ", in Kafka's *Handbuch*, op. cit. (Munich, 1922). An excellent monograph, containing over 320 bibliographical citations and many illustrations. The chapter devoted to " Religion und Mythus " is particularly worth noting.

[27] Cf. Wundt, *Elemente der Völkerpsychologie* (Leipzig, 1912). Authorized English translation by E. L. Schaub : *Elements of Folk Psychology* (London, 1916).

[28] These methods are to be seen applied with varying success in almost all modern works dealing with the psychology of religion. Particularly noteworthy are the methods which have been adopted by Starbuck, Ribot, and Leuba. Cf. Dr. Karl Girgensohn's *Der seelische Aufbau des religiösen Erlebens*, etc. (Leipzig, 1921). This

book is based on the method of the questionnaire. The results are exceedingly slight.

[29] Georg Wobbermin, *Religion, die Methoden der religions-psychologischen Arbeit* (Berlin and Vienna, 1921). This is included in E. Abderhalden's *Handbuch*. The author critically examines the methods adopted by Stanley Hall and Starbuck, and the modified methods of Pfenningsdorf and H. Lehmann, and the principles and methods of Flournoy, Leuba, James, and Wundt. He also comments upon the ideas contained in Maier's *Psychologie des emotionalen Denkens* (Tübingen, 1908), in connection with emotional thought, and criticizes generally the methods of psycho-analysis in favour with the Freudians, and particularly that of Reik, of which I have given a short account. Wobbermin's monograph concludes with an account of the psychological structure of the religious consciousness. The central conception of this writer is the predomination in the religious consciousness of the desire to possess absolute truth; and a comprehensive theory ought to take into consideration this predominating desire.

[30] J. Huby, *La Conversion* (Paris, 1919), p. 94. This small book makes mention of several converts.

[31] Monsignore Mario Sturzo, "La psicologia della conversione" in the *Rivista di Filosofia neoscolastica*, 1915, p. 546. The author in this article considers that conversion consists in an active unification of the personality, determined by the unexpected outbreak of disturbances of the emotional life. Before conversion the inclinations are anonymous or ascribed to restlessness. He believes that there are psychodynamic moments. The author admits the instantaneity (a disease or a miracle?) of conversion, analogous to vocation. He also admits the elaborations of the subconscious mind, but indicates the way in which the convert fights against conversion and subsequently arrives at 'assent' (or a change of the will). The assent is conscious and voluntary. This is the author's theory, which is contrary to that of Mainage, who considers that the transcendant 'pulls' the convert irresistibly. By thus reasoning, Mainage puts conversion outside of psychology.

In a lecture delivered on 6th March, 1922, on "Conversions", Monsignore Mario Sturzo defined conversion as the passage from an orientation of life believed to be false and vicious to an orientation of life thought true and honest. Monsignore Sturzo here shows himself to be opposed to James's theory of the subconscious. Conversion, for him, is the harmonizing of the relative with the absolute, and in all conversions there is a spiritual battle between the relative and the absolute. Conversion for Monsignore Sturzo is the most perfect vindication of the finality of the world. The ultimate end of conversion is holiness, which is the supremest harmony between men and purposes, and is the nearest approach to the Absolute. The conversions which are instantaneous show most clearly the finger of God, the slow ones show most clearly the weight of man.

[32] Upon this is based the psychology of religion, and this was my contention in my lecture on " Conversion " of March, 1921. See the epitome contained in *Bylichnis* for February, 1921. In an editorial article, which appeared in the *Civiltà Cattolica*, 16th April, 1921, the writer, P. Barbèra, makes various criticisms on my lecture. The first is that I had exceeded the bounds of biology and had advanced into the sphere of rationalistic philosophy. To this one may reply that modern psychology is not purely descriptive, but is also explanatory. The writer insists upon the action of ' grace ', and this he declares to be present not only in all conversions, but in all the moral crises of the conscience, in whatever religion the subject believes; and in this connection the writer advises me to read the theological treatises upon ' grace ' and a study of it by Cardinal Billot, " La Providence de Dieu et le nombre infini d'hommes en dehors de la voie normale du salut ", which appeared in the *Études*, Paris, 20th August and 5th December, 1920. Evidently he advises me to digress widely! No psychologist can be a competent theologian. The critic of the *Civiltà Cattolica* defends the prerogative of ' grace ', denying that it is, psychologically speaking, a passive phenomenon, and affirming that even in instantaneous conversions the phenomenon is more active than ever. The question is an old one, and one that I know and would gladly have avoided. But there is a debate among the Catholics themselves ; some of them believe in a ' grace ' that works in obscurity, without the subject becoming aware of its antecedents, and others in a ' grace ' whose work in the individual is followed in all its phases by the subject's consciousness. Psychology does not criticize ' grace ' as Blondel does, nor does it affirm that God is the creation of our will. But neither does it psychologize upon God. Modern religious psychology limits itself to the consideration of the psychology of man when he experiences ' grace ' and God.

There have been attempts at a scientific study of ' grace '. Maine de Biran attempted the application of the introspective method to theology. But Maine de Biran himself concluded that it is the organic condition which determines our well-being or its opposite, and that the soul cannot escape from such determinism, and thus may be troubled. May ' grace ', perhaps, even act through the physical and the moral dispositions as its intermediaries ? According to this author : " We are dependent on the organism for the reception of superior light, and for the acquisition of truth ;

as we are dependent upon the good formation of our eyes for seeing the objective light." In short, the divine and the diabolical are not the objects of direct experience. Maine de Biran, disappointed in his hopes, at last abandoned the method from which he had such high expectations.

Monsignor Bougaud is one of the chief representatives of intimate apologetics applied to dogma. Joseph de Maistre preceded him. It has been said that dogmas are discovered in us not as in fire . . . but as in a reflection (*réflet*). We have them sometimes as a presentiment and sometimes as a reality (de Maistre). It is easy to conceive of a Christian soul finding Christianity within itself ; but does the non-Christian soul also find it there ? Bougaud replies it can ; but this is inadmissible. These questions are dealt with in Xavier Moisant's *Dieu : l'expérience en métaphysique*, op. cit. This writer concludes that theodicy obtains no light from psychological experiences. According to the opinion of Lachelier in *Du fondement de l'induction* (Paris, 1896), neither ' grace ' nor dogma are matters of experience. The Deity is not an object of normal intuition or of direct affirmation. The method of immanence cannot serve here. We have not within ourselves any sufficient reason for our existence, or the supreme principle of moral law which attaches us to life, or the object of felicity to which we aspire : thus Moisant. The psychologist confronted even by such negations as these, feels himself an agnostic.

For the understanding of the so-called ' pure affective state ' and also on the subject of the subconscious mind, the reader is recommended to read Maine de Biran's *Memoire sur les perceptions obscures suivi de la discussion avec Royer Collard sur l'existence d'un état purement affectif et de trois notes inédites* (Paris, 1920).

[33] On this subject the reader may consult an old book : *Sacre metamorfosi o vero conversioni segnalate d'Idolotri, Turchi, Ebrei, e Eretici convertiti alla Fede cattolica et altri passati da' Peccati, e dal secolo, alla Penitenza et alla Religione, cavate da diversi scrittori antichi e moderni*, per Girolamo Bascape, Milanese, Prete della congregazione dell' Oratorio di S. Filippo Neri, della città di Napoli. In Napoli M.DC.LXXXII. Per Novello De Bonis stampatore arcivescovile, con licenza dei superiori.

[34] Biography and hagiography present a sufficiently untrustworthy source of historical knowledge. The saints on one side only are historical ; on the other side they are legendary. Cf. Delehaye's *Le leggende agiografiche*, Italian translation (Florence, 1906) ; also P. Santyves, *Les Saints successeurs des Dieux* (Paris, 1907). At the present time the Library, *Les Saints*, inaugurated by H. Joly, is a serious step in the right direction.

[35] Sante de Sanctis, " Psicologia della vocazione," in the *Rivista di Psicologia* (vol. xv, Bologna, 1919). In this article I refer

particularly to the selection of a profession; in the beginning
I also deal with the subject of religious vocation.

³⁶ Professor James H. Leuba, whose article published in 1902
has already been mentioned, has occupied himself to a great
extent with religious phenomena. His doctor's thesis, " Studies
in the Psychology of Religious Phenomena—Conversion ", in the
Amer. Journal of Psychology (vol. vii, 1896), is a study of Christian
conversion. Leuba examines the origin of religious phenomena,
in the customs and the beliefs of primitive peoples, and in its
manifestations in infantile life. His books display a wealth of
anthropological and sociological as well as psychological
knowledge. All his writings seek to establish a scientific theory
of religion.

Leuba's scope extends beyond the limts of religious psychology
as defined by Flournoy. Leuba in fact contends that the transcendental should be an object of psychological study, on a par
with the experiences of salvation and of faith in God. To sum up,
Leuba is a ' psychologist ' in the sense of one who maintains the
explicability of everything by psychology; moreover, according
to him, sociology merges into psychology.

See also Leuba's *The Belief in God and Immortality* (1916),
and more recently his *Psychology of Religious Mysticism* (London,
1925), in the Library of Psychology, Philosophy, and Scientific
Method.

At the end of the French translation of Leuba's *A Psychological Study of Religion* (*La psychologie des phenomenes religieux*,
Paris, 1914) is a bibliographical note on Leuba's publications on
religious psychology. The quotations from Leuba which are
found interspersed in the present book, do not refer only to the
French edition, but include citations from other of his writings,
and especially from the report of the Sixth International Congress
of Psychology at Geneva, in 1909.

³⁷ Kurt Rothe, *Auf dem Heimwege: Beiträge zur Seelenkunde
und Seelenpflege unserer suchenden Zeitgenossen* (Paderborn,
1921). This is a most important lecture, both on account of its
bibliography and of its fine psychological analyses and its practical
advice.

³⁸ The present book had already been written several months
when I read that most interesting work of Henri Delacroix,
La Religion et la foi (Paris, 1922). The tenth chapter of Book III
of this work deals particularly with the theme of Conversion. The
author gives a general treatment of this subject and considers
the phenomenon in all its various psychological aspects, and ends
by giving (on page 341) the classic scheme of conversion in all its
phases. The task to which I address myself is considerably
more modest. However, the views of this author do not implicitly

T

exclude my own, nor vice versa. Delacroix opposed the
'affectivists'; but on that point I find myself only partly in
agreement with him.

CHAPTER II

[1] J. M. Baldwin, in the *Dictionary of Philosophy and Psychology*
(New York, 1911), vol. i, on page 232, writes that in Logic the
term Conversion is employed to denote "the process by which,
from a given proposition called the Convertend, there is educed
or inferred another proposition, called the Converse, in quality
the same as the original proposition, and having for its subject the
predicate, and for its predicate the subject of the original
proposition".

In regard to Baldwin's Theory of Memory, the reader should
see the comprehensive work of this author : *Thought and Things*
(London and New York, 1906-9).

[2] Sigmund Freud, *Vorlesungen zur Einführung in die
Psychoanalyse*, part iii, Allg. Neurosenlehre (Leipzig and Vienna,
1918). [English translation, *Introductory Lectures on Psycho-
analysis*, London, 1922.]

[3] This, and other quotations from Seneca, I have taken from
Martha, *Les Moralistes sous l'Empire Romain—Philosophes et
poetes* (Paris, 1866).

[4] L. Papus, *Traité élémentaire de Science occulte* (Paris, 1903),
in the seventh edition on page 495, et seq., where the author
gives an account of his conversion.

[5] James, *Varieties of Religious Experience*, A study in human
nature ; being the Gifford Lectures on Natural Religion (London,
1903).

[6] J. Rouges de Fursac, *Un Mouvement mystique contemporain.
Le reveil religieux du Pays de Galles (1904-1905)* (Paris, 1907). The
author gives an account of the observations he made during his
special visit to England in 1906 in order to study the Welsh
Revivalist Movement initiated at Loughor by a student named
Evan Roberts. This was the Revival movement which resulted in
a harvest of some 100,000 conversions. The author deals with the
conversions in the second part of the book, on page 66 et seq. A short
chapter of special interest to the alienist is the one which begins
on page 121. The book, as a whole, is of limited interest,
particularly in relation to the psychology of religion. The author
says that the conversions were chiefly temporary (he computes
these at 95 per cent), and that the subjects, who were largely
drunkards, converted during the Revivals, are not to be counted

as true converts.   He does not deny the value of the Revivals
on this account.   In fact, these Revivalist Meetings proved useful
for the general level of morality, individually and socially, because
the conversions produced a marked effect upon the curve of crime
and of alcoholic psychoses throughout Wales.

⁷ " Giosuè Borsi e il Cardinal Maffi," an article by Soter in
Bilychnis, a monthly review of religious studies (Rome, 1920),
No. 10, p. 253.

The author denies that Borsi's case is to be regarded as a conversion proper ; it was rather a gradual realization of his true
self.   Borsi himself, in his *Confessioni a Giulia*, dated
6th December, 1912, writes : " Everything in the world is
established by eternal law ; and the clear recognition of this
truth I owe to you.   I waited for you, with the inward conviction that you would dawn upon me one day, and that I should
know you at once as queen of my heart and arbiter of my destiny.
At certain moments I felt how much there was in this love of pre-
destination and of fate ; that there was something superior to my
small and futile human will.   Each wandering path where I was
lost led me back to you—always."   Substitute for ' Giulia ', God,
says the writer of the article, and the full meaning of Giosuè
Borsi's life will be apparent.   Borsi learned from his father to despise
money.   From the days of his childhood he gave promise of an
exceptionally quick intelligence and feeling.   The years between
1910 and 1914 were the years which tried Borsi.   The deaths of his
father, his sister, and of the little Dino were successive blows.
The material preoccupations of life began to weigh upon him.
Throughout the pages of his diary we can follow Borsi, step
by step, during his slow approach to God.   The gradual transition
from earthly to heavenly love was almost insensibly effected.
It was a truly progressive recognition of his own self.   " From
certain signs that I read in the book of the future, I thought I
should conquer," said Borsi, " but I did not imagine what this
victory was to cost me."   Cardinal Maffi was his great sustainer
during this ascent.   Borsi's first meeting with him took place on
the 19th December, 1914.   In his intercourse with the Cardinal,
all the conflicting elements of his nature became fused into a
superhuman harmony which flowed outwards, freely and
triumphantly, in that perfected Christianity which death has
glorified.

The *Civiltà Cattolica* (No. 1700, 16th April, 1921) contains a
critical analysis of Borsi's *Confessioni a Giulia* by Pietro Misciatelli
" In these pages ", says the reviewer, " the steps of the purification
can be clearly seen passing slowly and haltingly from the debase-
ment of the lower passions, towards the more human, the nobler,
and holier emotions of family love."

[8] Alphonse Primot, *La Psychologie d'une conversion du positivisme au spiritualisme* (Paris, 1914). I have only been able to find the first volume of this work.

[9] The number of accounts, biographical and autobiographical, of conversions is infinite. I do not intend to make a list of them here. I quote almost at random : C. J. Chevé's *Dictionnaire des conversions* (Paris, 1866). Andreas Räss, *Die Convertiten seit der Reformation nach ihrem Leben und aus ihren Schriften dargestellt* (Freiburg, i. B. 1866 and 1880), a work in 13 volumes, Catholic and distinctly apologist in tone, but rich in information. Alban Stolz, *Fügung und Führung Konvertitenbilder*, edited by Dr. Julius Mayer (Freiburg, i. B. 1912). In this book an account is given of the German converts of the first half of the nineteenth century. David August Rosenthal, *Convertitenbilder aus dem neunzehnten Jahrhundert* (Schaffhausen, 1866). There is a more recent edition of this work, published in Regensburg in 1889, and also two supplements published in Regensburg in 1902, which give accounts of other conversions of the nineteenth century. On the subject of German conversions, Gisbert Menge's book, *Die Wiedervereinigung im Glauben* (Freiburg, 1914). The first volume, *Die Glaubenseinheit*, especially chapter xi, should be noted.

On the subject of French conversions, the best of all descriptions are among the writings of Père Mainage, who is responsible for the Paris *Journal des jeunes*. In the issue of that paper for 25th May, 1920, there is an article by Noble on the conversion of Ernest Psichari, whose life has also been written by Henri Massis. See also A. M. Goichon, *Ernest Psichari, d'après des documents inédites* (Paris, 1921).

Ernest Psichari, who was the nephew of Ernest Renan, was one of the soldier-poets who fell in the war. He became a convert to Catholicism slowly, and without any crisis. He wrote a private journal which was published under the title of *Les voix qui crient dans le désert* (Paris, 1920), and another book called the *Voyage du Centurion*, which has been translated into Italian.

A recent book which deals with modern French conversions is one edited by Father Mainage entitled: *Nos convertis*; of this there is an Italian translation, *Come ci siamo convertiti*. It contains autobiographical descriptions by various converts : André de Bavier, Pierre de Lescure, Puel de Lobel, Dumesnil, Claudel, and many others, collected by Father Mainage. The Italian translation, which contains a preface written by Cardinal Pietro Maffi, is by Antonio Masini : Turin. The book bears no date, but the preface is dated 1918.

In Italian also there have been a few monographs on converts, either original or translations. An instance is Semeria's *Gente che torna, gente che si muove, gente che si avvia* (Genoa, 1901) ; in this little book the author deals with the æsthetic conversions of Huysmans, Paul Bourget, François Coppée, Jules Lemaître, and Adolph Retté. (Certain of these conversions were not believed to be genuine by the reformist Catholics of the period.) There is an Italian version of Adolph Retté's account of his conversion, with a preface by François Coppée, called *Dal diavolo a Dio*, L. Cassis's translation (Treviso, 1908). There is also an Italian translation of Ruville, called *Il Mio Ritorno*.

[10] Stanley Hall, *Adolescence: and its Relations*, etc. (New York, 1904), vol. ii. A most interesting book on account of the statistics to which it refers.

D. L. Moody and M. S. Kees admit the greater frequency of conversions between the ages of 10 and 20 years ; other authorities, after the age of 15. Cf. Stanley Hall, vol. ii, p. 288 et seq., and the table on p. 290, giving the evidence in support of the greater frequency, which according to him occurs in both sexes between the ages of 11 and 23 years. The affirmation of religious consciousness, according to George A. Coe, *The Spiritual Life* (New York, 1920), occurs as follows : At 13 the first premonition, at 17 the second, at 20 the maximum of intensity occurs. Boys and girls are but slightly influenced by religion in childhood ; before the age of 12 religion is a mere matter of form according to Lancaster. Cf. Stanley Hall, p. 292, vol. ii, where the author discusses at length the researches of Starbuck.

See also Havelock Ellis's *Man and Woman*, which was translated into Italian by C. Del Soldato from the fourth English edition, as vol. xxiv, of the *Indagine moderna* series (undated). It contains diagrams of the frequency of conversions from the ages of 6 to 25 years, gathered from the American authors, particularly Starbuck.

[11] Stanley Hall, op. cit., vol. ii, p. 331.

[12] It is observed that the psycho-sexual crisis of puberty corresponds naturally to the development of the genital organs and functions. The psycho-sexual crisis shows itself in its various phases in schools and colleges, where the direct expression of normal sexuality is inhibited. The φιλία of the Hellenic world, the Socratic love which united youths in the groves and in the porticos of the gymnasia are classical instances. ' Flaming love ', which is mostly homo-sexual, is one of the sorrows of adolescence and boyhood, and is not seldom the cause of the homo-sexual tendencies of later youth. A useful contribution to this subject is the well-documented work of Obici and Marchesini, *Le Amicizie di Collegio*.

For the biosexual development of the adolescent, cf. Stanley Hall, op. cit., vol. i, chapter 6.

[13] Everyone, in and out of Italy, knows the work of Cesare

Lombroso, of Marro, and of Ferriani, on criminality in adolescence. Cf. Stanley Hall, op. cit., vol. i, chap. 5; and Sante De Sanctis, *Patologia e profilassi mentale* (Milan, undated). See Appendix; Relazione intorno alla profilassi della delinquenza dei minorenni," published 1910.

This is not the place to demonstrate the frequency of criminality in the adolescent period. It is a fruitful subject on which a voluminous literature exists, extending from past decades up to the present. I must content myself with mention of two articles which give a résumé of the subject : one by Alfredo Spallanzani " Della delinquenza dei minorenni in Italia negli anni 1891–1917 secondo le statistiche giudiziarie." The other is by Dr. Fanny Dalmazzo, " L'Inghilterra e il problema della precoce delinquenza." Both appeared in the August and September numbers of the review *La scuola positiva*, edited by Enrico Ferri and Eugenio Florian (Milan, 1921).

[14] In a table of Starbuck's, republished in F. Giese's article, " Allgemeine Kinderpsychologie ", in Kafka's *Handbuch*, op. cit., an instructive summary of the motives which give rise to conversions is given :—

		Women. %	Men. %
1.	Fear of death or damnation	14	14
2.	Other egocentric motives	5	7
3.	Altruistic motives	6	4
4.	Tendency towards ethical ideals	15	20
5.	Remorse of conscience, sense of guilt, etc.	15	18
6.	Influence of teaching	11	8
7.	Example, imitation, etc.	14	12
8.	Social environment, moral pressure, etc.	20	17

On analysis this shows :—

	Women	Men
1 + 2 Egocentric motives	19	21
3 + 4 Altruistic motives	21	24
1 — 5 Subjective forces	55	63
6 — 8 Objective forces	45	37

[15] In Russia the persecutions of the Bolsheviks has brought about a revival of the spirit of martyrdom in religion. This result has at least been noticeable in the behaviour of the Metropolitan Benjamin of Leningrad and of the late Patriarch Tikhon of Moscow. In Germany, after the collapse of the war, a notable religious re-awakening has been observed. This has been displayed by the multiplication of new sects, and their rapid, if ephemeral, success, by the mystic colour of certain scientific and political movements, and also by the remarkable number of

conversions from Protestantism to Catholicism. In Germany the number of Protestants—or more strictly, non-Catholics—becoming Catholics in a decade averages about five per cent of the total non-Catholic population, which is nearly thirty-nine millions. The passage from Catholicism to Protestantism, it is true, amounts to eight per cent, but this is reckoned on the much smaller Catholic population of twenty millions. However, as the Catholic writers have pointed out, many factors operate on a religious minority living amongst a population 61 per cent of whom belong to a different religious faith. Among other contributory causes is divorce, which is legally recognized for Protestants, but not for those of the Catholic religion.

I am indebted to Monsignor Mann, Director of the Collegio Beda in Rome, for the information that in England almost every family of the upper middle class has one Catholic (converted) member. In England mass-conversion has never been customary, but individual conversions are always occurring. In 1921 there were 13,000 English conversions *to* Catholicism. During that year almost no conversions *from* Catholicism were made. Counter-conversions in England are of exceptionally rare occurrence, and are due, if ever, to marriages with Protestants, etc.

The data on the noteworthy movement towards Catholicism in the United States of America are to be found in the American review, *The Missionary* (cf. numbers for May, June, and October, 1921), and in the recent work of P. E. J. Mannix, *The American Convert Movement* (New York, 1923).

¹⁶ *Fioretti del glorioso messere Sancto Francesco e dei suoi frati* (Sansoni, Florence, 1918), chapter 26 and chapter 1.

¹⁷ See Pietro Misciatelli, *Mistici Senesi* (Siena, 1911).

¹⁸ The sermons of Savonarola produced multitudes of converts. Bettuccio, a Florentine full of impetuosity, quarrelsome, a corrupt libertine, and a partisan of the Arrabiati faction against the Piagnoni, after much urging went to the Cathedral to pray. At once he felt Savonarola's eyes fixed upon him. Much shaken, he went off to a solitary place and " for the first time in my life I felt my mind accuse itself ". He spent a long time in meditation, went home, and felt himself entirely changed. From that moment his habits altered. He attended the sermons at San Marco. He had a severe contest with his old companions, and a harder struggle against his passions. At length he felt sure of himself, and went and knelt before Savonarola. The great preacher refused to accept him. He told him to undergo still more experiences. So Bettuccio continued the struggle against his passions, though sometimes he succumbed. Then at last he took Dominican orders on 7th November, 1495, and became Fra Benedetto. His autobiographical poem tells the story of his conversion. After the

death of Savonarola, Fra Benedetto killed a man and was sent to prison, but did penance. Cf. *La storia di Girolamo Savonarola e de' suoi tempi*, by Pasquale Villari (new and augmented edition, with the author's corrections; third impression, in 2 vols., Florence, 1910).

[19] E. Bonajuti, S. *Agostino* in " Profili di Formiggini ", No. 44 (Rome, 1917), to which P. N. Concetti's S. *Agostino* is a polemic reply (Rome, Scuola tipografica Salesiana, 1919). I had reference to this little book in my citation.

[20] *Fioretti di S. Francesco*, op. cit., p. 203.

[21] William James has devoted a penetrating critique to the *pari de Pascal*. My reference is to the French translation, *La volonté de Croire* (Paris, 1916), page 25.

[22] Peter van der Meer de Walcheren, *Journal d'un Converti*, 1917, quoted in Mainage's work.

[23] Mink-Jullien, *Les voies de Dieu* (1917) (cited in Mainage, op. cit.).

[24] Don Illemo Camelli, *Dal Socialismo al Sacerdozio* (6th edition, Brescia, 1921). An unpretentious little book in which the author lays more stress on his interior evolution than upon the external facts that motivated it ; especially interesting for the psychologist on that account. Camelli, who was a painter, had always been an emotional enthusiast, and, from his boyhood, had been a mystic Socialist ; he was distrustful of the intellectuals, full of humanitarian faith, and ready for self-sacrifice. His passage over to the Catholic religion was slow, and helped by his early family training. He had his crises of sensuality ; he loved, but was not given to libertinage, so that he conserved a tremendous amount of psychic energy, which enabled him to perform work as an artist, a Socialist, and a Christian mystic. The disillusions of party politics, the need for authoritative guidance, a long and painful illness, and the death of a friend permitted him to feel, on several occasions through visions of Nature and of art, the divine ' touch ', and to hear within him a voice, ' distinct and strong ', which replied to his repeated questioning : " When thou has lost all, thou shalt find all." (This was an imaginary audition, not an auditory hallucination.) He was abandoned by the woman he loved, and his solitude and moral depression led him almost to the point of suicide. Then the company of two deeply religious persons, a dream, and the influence of the Barnabite Father Tommaso Zoia led him to take the sacrament. Finally, at the age of 29, in 1905, he was ordained a priest.

[25] E. Leseur, *Journal et pensées de chaque jour* (Paris, 1917).

[26] Giovanni Papini, *Lettera a Mazzucconi* ; published in the daily press. I shall have occasion to mention Papini again in the notes to Chapter IV.

²⁷ Frederick Joseph Kinsman, former Bishop of the American Episcopalian Church at Delaware, some years ago became a convert to Catholicism. His book, describing his conversion, *Salve Mater* (New York and London, 1920), at once went into two editions, one in February, the other in May. In his preface he states that he has in no way altered his principles, but only changed the method of their application. He also admits that ever since his conversion his personal feeling towards the Anglican Communion is one of profound gratitude. He declares that after he had joined the church of Rome, the past appeared to him as through a veil, making it difficult for him to recall to memory what he had formerly felt (see chapter x). In chapter xiv he deals with the psychology of his conversion, and emphasizes the fact that the disappearance of illusions and the removal of prejudices do not constitute a conversion. He remarks that certain of his changes of opinion which he can remember occurred not only when he had no intention of relinquishing this position in the American Episcopalian Church, but were co-existent with the desire he felt to retain it. He relates that his opinions in regard to the Catholic religion passed through four stages : first, in which he felt that, after all, it was 'not so bad '; second, that it was really a good thing; third, that it was the best thing he knew; and lastly, that it was the Church. It was only when he had arrived at the last conviction that the conversion was genuine. The third stage, however, required a change of belief which consisted in a recognition of the supremacy of the Catholic Church and of the ' exigency of the Papal claim '. He did not declare these convictions at the time for several reasons. He was Bishop of Delaware, and he wanted to wait and debate the grounds of his opinions. Then for a time he felt that there were only two alternatives : Agnosticism or the Church of Rome. Then he saw that Christianity divided against itself was distasteful and paralyzing. This conviction grew clearer and more forcible day by day. All those thoughts, which had at first seemed confused, became gradually disentangled and co-ordinated, and assumed their due proportions. When he regarded the world he now perceived the semblance of a new order of things. He now recognized the absurdity of individual reason appraising, understanding, or deciding anything. Some old opinions seemed purposeless or mad, although they acquired a new value, as fitting into place in relationship to things as a whole. As far as he could actually remember, his only sensation was that of contentment. He declared that he had not looked for personal happiness, or peace, or advantage. What he desired was to become identified with the Catholic Church, to which his life was dedicated. Having discovered that which he believed to be the true Ark of Salvation,

any personal desire was immediately and wholly satisfied. He regarded his life of activity as being in all probability over for ever ; but that he would have to disregard. It was certainly an immense relief to abandon the attempts he had been making to reform the Church—a necessary aim when he held his former views—and instead, simply to submit to being himself reformed by the Church. That, as he said, seemed to him to be a much more rational way in which to regard things.

Newman said it was not Rome, but Oxford, that had made him a Catholic. Kinsman says the same thing, substituting for Oxford St. Paul's School, where he was educated, and where the foundations of his religious development and religious instincts had already been firmly laid. Newman's words in *Loss and Gain* are quoted by the writer, as explaining how his final doubts were resolved regarding the Mother Church, at what was probably the true moment of his conversion : " What is the Communion of Saints ? " It was then that there burst from his lips the invocation to this Mother All-Powerful, as he hastened his steps with almost unseemly eagerness on the upward path.

[28] St. Augustine : " *Ego vero Evangelio non crederem, nisi me Catholicae Ecclesiae commoveret auctoritas* " (*Contra Man.*, Ep. V).

[29] The conversion of Manzoni's hero " Innominato ", was rapid. But it was a typically ' progressive ' process, and decidedly not ' fulminant ' in type. The case is of particular interest since we can observe in it the determining motive of powerful moral needs. On closely studying the process of this conversion, it is easy to perceive its unconscious elements ; but what stands out still more noticeably is the element of volition. Manzoni's " Innominato " was a man of 60, a rich noble who had been exiled from Milan. He came back to the state as a small squire, and established himself on the borders in a ruined castle as an outlaw and the protector of bandits ; he was ruthless, intolerant of the law, impulsive, daring, determined. When Don Roderigo came to Castellaccio to propose to him the affair of Lucia, Innominato, it is true, at once agreed to help him, but Manzoni explains that " no sooner was he (Innominato) alone, than he was—I could hardly say—penitent, but angry at having given his word. He had for some time past been conscious of a feeling of something which was akin to remorse and of a sensation of a sort of unworthiness about his villainies . . . A kind of repugnance, like that which he had felt about his first crimes, but which he had overcome, had come back again." After a night of terrible interior conflict, Innominato went to Cardinal Federigo. It is here that Manzoni makes the important observation : " Innominato was as if transported outside of himself by the overpowering force of an inexplicable frenzy, rather

than led by a determined purpose." After some instants of silent expectation, and after the Cardinal's words, Innominato cried out : " God ! God ! God ! If I could but see Him : if I could only feel Him. Where is this God . . . ? " And the embrace followed by these words : " God is great, God is good. Now I know, now I understand . . . and I feel such joy as I have never felt before in all my vile existence." The crisis had come, a definite salvation ; the *mutatio dexterae excelsi*. And the conversion was effectuated under the pressure of a moral necessity.

[30] Johannes Jœrgensen, *Dal Pelago alla riva*. (The Italian translation to which I here refer contains a preface by A. Gemelli.) (Mantua, 1919).

[31] Monsignor Robert Hugh Benson, *The Confessions of a Convert*. I quote from the French translation by Theodore de Wyzewa (Paris, 1914). The words quoted are from Benson. The book itself should be read to convince readers of the truth of what has been stated in the text. The conversion of Robert Hugh Benson is unquestionably an instance of the typically intellectual conversion, with which—in the present work—I have not been concerned. No one who has read these confessions, however, could fail to appreciate that this intellectual also possessed an ardent and deeply mystical soul. He was intensely sensitive to music, which was, he says, the single thread, at one period of his life, which bound him to the supernatural ; the little religion which he then had came wholly through a love of art. While awaiting his ordination as an Anglican clergyman, after making a general confession, he fell into a sort of beatific ecstacy. Subsequently he took up work, with intense enthusiasm, in an East London parish.

[32] Reports and publications of the Geneva Psychological Congress, op. cit., chap. i, p. 712.

CHAPTER III

[1] Kurt Rothe, *Auf dem Heimwege*, op. cit. This author distinguishes seven stages in the process. *First stage* : The searcher (*Suchende*) recognizes that he has not previously entertained the right views regarding the Catholic Church, and begins to know Catholic truths by means of books, artistic imagination, social intercourse, and so forth, which chance (or, as this author puts it, ' grace ') throws in his way. *Second stage* : He begins to have a clearer perception of the edifice of faith and becomes aware of its beauty from literature, especially religious works. *Third stage* : He begins to realize that the doctrines of

the Church are obviously worthy of serious examination, and that their foundations are more firmly based than anything else. *Fourth stage* : He tries, by way of experiment, to live like a Catholic, and recognizes the superiority of the Catholic faith in his struggle to educate his habits. *Fifth stage* : He comes to know the unity and the uniqueness of the Holy Church for humanity and for himself. *Sixth stage* : Human and external difficulties which he has to encounter, and also involuntary revulsions from the exigencies of the Church, make the inquirer conscious of a painful uncertainty. *Seventh stage* : After severe struggles, his prayers finally open for him the ' path to grace ', and the inquirer has completed his conversion.

The author devotes special attention to each of these stages. The succeeding chapters of the book will show the difference between our own views and those of Rothe. Meanwhile, the reader will note that he is chiefly concerned with the intellectual process of conversion, while admitting—as we ourselves admit—the superiority of the *conversio cordis* over that of the *conversio mentis*.

² The writer Valois passed from a militant anarchy to an ever serener view of life by a slow interior evolution, through the influence of his external life, rich in experiences of many countries and peoples. After his happy marriage and after he had obtained an appointment of modest security, he felt a revival of the faith of his forefathers. The sanctity of motherhood, as he saw it revealed in his own family, suggested to him the conception of a diviner motherhood, keeping eternal vigil over mankind. He felt, at length, the insufficiency of demagogic conceptions inadequate to the deepest needs of human life. And so, shortly after his thirtieth year, his inner life, like his exterior life, was put in order, and he became a practising Catholic. See Georges Valois, *D'un siècle à l'autre* (Paris, 1922).

³ J. H. Leuba, op. cit., in the bibliography to Chapter I.

⁴ Father Mainage, *Psychologie de la Conversion*, op. cit.

⁵ F. H. W. Myers, *Human Personality and its Survival of Bodily Death* (London, 1909) (Italian translation : *La personalità umana e la sua sopravvivenza*, Rome, 1909).

⁶ All the works of Sigmund Freud contain expositions of his views on the theory of the Unconscious. See : *Vorlesungen zur Einführung in die Psychoanalyse* (*Introductory Lectures on Psycho-analysis*, London, 1922). Also " Das Unbewusste " in the *Intern. Zeitschrift für Ärztliche Psychoanalyse*, 1915. See also note 23 to Chapter I.

It is unnecessary here to restate the Freudian theory of the Unconscious. I need only refer to the distinction which is made between " unconscious representations " and " latent memories ". The Freudians, in order to prove the psychic existence of the unconscious, assert that the actions, for instance, which follow suggestion, and the so-called unconscious representations in general, unlike latent memories, give proof of the subjective existence of the unconscious. Thus, according to them, unconscious representations have a certain degree of independence of the conscious ego, while latent memory does not display itself as a subjective state. We do not feel the need of this distinction. See on the subject of this discussion Dr. Eduard Weiss, " Alcuni concetti fondamentali della psicoanalisi " in the *Rivista Sperimentale di Freniatria*, vol. xlv, Nos. 3 and 4.

Weiss does not appear to make any distinction between what I call the *subconscious* and what the Freudians call the *unconscious* (*Unbewusste*), considering it a question of terminology. Here an explanation becomes imperative. It is well known that the psychoanalysts themselves admit of two kinds of unconscious ; the preconscious, or *Vorbewusste*, which is capable of becoming conscious, and the true unconscious, or *Unbewusste*, which is incapable of becoming conscious, except by passing through the transitional sphere of the preconscious. This distinction serves the pseudo-Freudians as a description of psychic dynamics. We disregard any such distinction, and therefore do not conform to what is popularly called the ' topical ' point of view of psycho-analysis ; we adhere to the term subconscious, or *Unterbewusste*, in spite of the objections of the psycho-analysts, including Freud. Subconscious is a term which not only indicates the level of consciousness and implies the possibility of all the contents of the subconscious mind eventually becoming conscious in their turn (which clearly is not so in the case of the unconscious in our sense) ; but at the same time the term subconscious suggests the conception of the primacy of the activity of consciousness. In fact, for us, consciousness is the recognition of old and new situations, or of former conscious or subconscious experiences ; it is the choice, the acceptance, and the realization of material adapted to immediate or distant aims.

But the term subconscious also possesses for us another merit. It implies the idea that the conscious and the subconscious are indissolubly linked together, and are in continuous intercommunication. This conception finds strong support in the anatomy, histology, and physiology of the nervous system. The conscious and the subconscious—or as the others call it, the unconscious—are not two separate stores of contents, nor are they two different fields of action. Such a metaphysical conception can be both used and abused, but on a closer consideration it is necessary to be explicit.

The suggestion of a clear distinction between the conscious and the subconscious was first made by the French psychologists ;

it was then put forward more insistently by Myers in his theory of the " Subliminal Self " ; ultimately it was advocated by the Freudians. But if, in rare instances, the subconscious self may become so systematized as to constitute an ephemeral personality in the case of hysterical psychasthenics, nothing of the kind occurs among sane persons.   Of this we can convince ourselves, on the one hand, from the structure and nature of the central nervous system, and on the other hand, from the unprejudiced observation of facts.

Just as there is no discontinuity between the cortical centres of perception and those of memory—the one being the seat of the elaborations of conscious actuality, the other of the personal subconscious—so in the same way there is no break in the intimate connection between the neencephalon and the palencephalon—the one being the seat of personal experiences and the other of the subconscious mechanism.   We frequently see the subcortical and mesencephalic systems, which are to all appearances autonomous, influenced by the cortex, which either inhibits them or impels them to action.   On the other hand, in the appraisement of the dynamics of the unconscious, it must be borne in mind that the absence of a representation in conscious actuality may certainly imply its non-existence, though it may also be due to forgetting.   There is no way in which to prove that any given representation or idea was never at any time conscious. We are, it is true, profoundly ignorant respecting the relations between the conscious mind and the subconscious.   It can, however, be confidently stated that the psychic reflexes, in the sense of the Russian school, inform the entire psychic mass, whether actual or potential ; and that at least one portion of a given group of psychic reflexes passes into the subconscious and another portion into the conscious mind.

The term ' unconscious ', on the contrary, clearly implies a negation of such continuity of intercommunication and tends to emphasize the conception of an unconscious personality, in the pathological sense, or of the ' subliminal self ' of Myers.

In short, the term subconscious does not include the conception of a splitting of the personality ; and this is important, since, on the subject of pathological splitting of the personality—or depersonalization—there is much to be said.

On the other hand, between conscious and subconscious there is a perpetual current of intercommunication, even in dreams, as I believe I have already demonstrated.   It is clear, therefore, that my conception of the subconscious approaches that of *Sphäre* (*Schilder*) or of *Randbewusstsein*, rather than Freud's.

[7] Théodule Ribot, *L'évolution des idées générales* (Paris, 1897). English edition, *The Evolution of General Ideas* (London, 1899).

[8] Fr. Paulhan, " Sur le psychisme inconscient ", in the *Journal de Psychologie normale et path*, 1921. The author maintains that the processes of the unconscious are identical in character with the processes of consciousness.   There are then, feeling, ideation, intelligence, and activity of the unconscious, similar to the corresponding processes of the conscious.   The unconscious is neither a principle in metaphysics, nor a hidden personality, but is continuous with the life of the conscious mind, to which it is correlated.   They are two aspects of the same activity.   As it is not possible to explain the mechanism of a locomotive by what can be seen only, so it is impossible to explain psychological phenomena only in terms of conscious facts.

[9] Joseph Jastrow, *The Subconscious* (London, 1906) (French translation, Paris, 1908).

[10] Morton Prince, *The Dissociation of a Personality* (London and New York, 1906).   For fulminant conversions, see p. 353 et seq.   Cf. further Assagioli in *Psiche* (March and April, 1912), for an account of Morton Prince's theory of Co-consciousness.   On the Unconscious and Subconscious see Georges Dwelshauvers, *L'Inconscient* (Paris, 1916), and Ed. Abramowski, *Le subconscient normal* (Paris, 1918).

[11] Cf. W. Wundt, *Der Spiritismus, Eine sogenante wissenschaftliche Frage* (Leipzig, 1879), 2nd edition, in which he treats of the subconscious.

[12] Th. Ribot, " Le rôle latent des images motrices ", *Revue Phil.*, 1912.   On the subject of the subconscious mind, see also Ribot's *La vie inconsciente et les mouvements* (Paris, 1914).   See also Edward Abramowski, op. cit.   According to this author, kinæsthetic impressions remain when their related images have disappeared.   This is why they make themselves felt after they have been ' forgotten '.   For instance, the generic feeling makes us reject a wrong name when we have forgotten the right one.   The generic feelings are the emotive equivalents of forgotten representations.   Forgetting, therefore, is never complete.   By the side of the active memory there exists an affective memory.   The total mass of the past which is preserved in a state of cryptomnesia, forms the emotional basis of our personality or of the ego.   This theory is analogous to that of Ribot and Bergson.   There is no question of equivalence ;   the generic sentiments accompany even representations.

[13] In this relation Freud's *Psychopathologie des Alltagslebens* (Berlin, 1917) (English translation : *Psychopathology of Everyday Life*, London, 1914) should be read.
On the subject of *Lapsus* see also Freud's *Introductory Lectures on Psycho-Analysis*.

[14] Carl Gustav Jung, " La structure de l'inconscient," *Archives*

de Psychol. (Dec., 1916). A remarkable article, especially as regards psycho-pathology (assimilation of the unconscious). It contains much that is irrelevant to our subject. The author considers that the unconscious in normal individuals is linked up with consciousness ; it is only in the insane that the unconscious mind is autonomous. We are unconditionally in agreement with him here. The remarks of this author on the collective psyche are interesting. It includes, at the same time, the theory of Freud on the sexual impulse, and Adler's ' desire for power ' (*Machttheorie*) : Jung states that the reappearance of the collective psyche in the individual would result in the dissolution of the personality, or dementia præcox ; thus the personality seeks to free itself from the collective psyche.

Jung's scheme of the structure of the unconscious appears to be as follows :—

| Conscious Mind. | { Personal Impersonal | The ego (*das Ich*). |
| Unconscious Mind. | { Personal Impersonal | The subconscious ego (*das Selbst*). |

[Cf. also *Psychology of the Unconscious*, New York and London, 1916.]

It is not to be expected that modern works on the unconscious, or subconscious, should contain any new thing of importance. Often we find nothing whatever except a repetition of the old psychology of the instincts. The reader should on no account omit reading the fine work of Rudolf Brun : " Das Instinktproblem im Licht der modernen Biologie," in the *Archivio Svizzero di Neurologia e Psichiatria*, 1920, vol. vi, No. 1. Here the intuitions are dealt with, and also displacement (*Verschiebung*). There is also a pathological section and a very full bibliography. Besides this, William McDougall's " Instinct and the Unconscious " in the *British Journal of Psychology*, 1919, is important.. To be read also are the collected lectures of W. H. R. Rivers, *Instinct and the Unconscious* (Cambridge, 1920).

[15] See : Sante De Sanctis, *Psychologie des Traumes* (Munich, 1922), chapter iii.

[16] The theory of William James has been followed in America, Germany, and even in Italy. It was much advocated by the Modernists. The phenomena of conversion were regarded as resembling those which appear in a paranoiac delirium. They are powerful subconscious experiences which break out in the super-liminal sphere. See : " La Psicologia della Conversione ", the discussion on an article of Guido Ferrando in *Psiche* (April to June, inclusive, 1914). The American theory of the unconscious was criticized by A. Gemelli, op. cit., cf. chapters v and vi, in which

the author refers to and comments on the opinions of a number of others, including Delacroix, Maréchal, Munnynck, Poulain, and Pacheu.

[17] On the subject of the conversion of St. Paul, cf. the Acts of the Apostles xxii, 2 ; xxvi, 14. The bibliography on the conversion of St. Paul is fairly copious : from Renan to Sabatier, from Trezza to Monod, etc. For us it has only a limited interest. See, however, Carl von Weizsächer, *Das apostolische Zeitalter der christlichen Kirche* (Freiburg, 1886), (*Le Origini del cristianismo, ossia l'epoca apostolica.* Italian version, 1921, vol. i, Book 2, Chapter i).

It has been said that the famous conversion of the Apostle can be explained according to three alternatives : *First*, the atheistic or rationalist explanation, an hallucination (Trezza) or an epileptic attack (Lombroso and other alienists) ; *Second*, the naturalistic explanation, which is that Paul had already had more or less fleeting perceptions of his mutation, especially in the discussion with Stephen, and when he was present at his martyrdom ; that he was surprised by a thunderbolt, a nervous attack, or a sunstroke, at the very moment when his internal conflict was coming to a crisis ; *Third*, the evangelical explanation, which is that the fact can only be accounted for supernaturally, or, as Sabatier puts it, that it was a direct contact of the spirit of God with the spirit of man.

Certainly, according to the witnesses, the conversion of Paul was a fulminant crisis. The words of the Apostle himself exclude the possibility of his having already known the Christian faith, either through the apostles or otherwise. He denies that there had been any intervening human instrument in his conversion. But the words of Paul do not exclude his having had personal experiences. His violent hatred against the ' sect ' is to be taken as a strong argument to the contrary, because the existence of violence presupposes a conflict. Our theory is supported by the fact that Paul was present at the trial and martyrdom of Stephen, and that he was aware of the statement by the disciples respecting the resurrection of Jesus. One reflects that the fact of the Resurrection is the cardinal point on which hinge the faith and apostolate of St. Paul.

The psychologist, further, has to ask himself whether the evidence of the subject is always entirely trustworthy, even though it may be in good faith. The psychology of memory shows that it is possible in the giving of evidence to forget some things which, at one time, were clearly conscious. The passionate pursuit of a given aim narrows the field of memory ; the resplendent vision at the end deepens the obscurity surrounding small past events. On the other hand, it is obvious that the atheist explanation is nothing else than the phenomenon of Damascus interpreted in the sense, as we should term it, of an outward projection of the unconscious mind of Paul. But such an explanation does not account for the mutation which occurred in him. The naturalistic explanation is a very suitable one, but it needs to be strengthened by historical data. As to the third method of explanation, it in itself, in my opinion, does not actually contradict either the first or the second, because ' grace ' could work at certain special moments, and on certain occasions. This third method of explanation, however, transcends scientific research.

The reader may consult Giovanni Luzzi's *Fatti degli apostoli*, a translation and commentary (Florence, 1899), p. 149. The quotation from Renan is taken from that author's *Les Apôtres* (Paris, 1866), chapter x, p. 166 et. seq.

[18] The fact is related by St. Augustine himself in his *Confessions*. My allusion is taken from the account of L. Bertrand, *Saint Augustine* (Paris, 83rd edition), p. 24. The edition of which I have made most frequent use is that of Knöll, *Augustinus Confessiones* (Leipzig, 1920).

It is noteworthy that St. Augustine underwent a long period of pre-mutation which we trace back to the influence of his mother, Monica. We see, further, that in the autumn of 386 he retired to the villa of Verecondo at Cassiciaco to recover from an intestinal indisposition, and that there, in view of Monte Rosa, his conversional process matured. Cf. on this point, Alfaric, *L'Évolution intellectuelle de St. Augustin*, vol. i, *Du Manicheisme au neoplatonisme* (Paris, 1918).

[19] The words of St. Augustine are in chapter ii, n. 5, of the *Confessions*.

[20] For the conversion of St. Francis, cf. the various lives of the saint. I have before me at present that of Paul Sabatier, *La vie de S. François d'Assise* (Paris, ed. of 1920) ; Johannes Jœrgensen, *Vita di S. Francesco*, translation authorized by the author (Palermo, 1910), historical sources, ancient and modern, are dealt with in a long introduction. See also Gaetan Schnürer's *Francesco d'Assisi*, translated from the German by Prof. Angelo Mercati, Florence, illustrated, with brief notes ; B. C. D'Andermatt's *Vita di S. Francesco D'Assisi*, translated by Prof. Giovanni Cattaneo (Innsbruck, 1902) ; Leopold Chérancé's *S. Francesco di Assisi*, 3rd It. edition, translated from the French (Venice, 1917).

[21] A. Müller, *Luthers Werdegang bis zum Turmerlebnis* (Gotha, 1920), reviewed in *Bilychnis*, Rome, September, 1920. I am unwilling to believe, with Denifle, that Luther was lying, but it seems to me clear that the meaning of the *Justitia Dei* had already been sought for and anxiously awaited by Luther. In the

Turmerlebnis there is probably an analogy to what is found in a mnemonic effort—as in the search for a name, a word, or a date—or an intellectual effort as in the solution of a problem or the discovery of an answer to an objection.

Delacroix, in his recent book, op. cit., speaks of Luther in chapter iii of book i. On p. 205 et seq. the author treats of the dogmatic evolution of the reformer. But even from this aspect the conversion of Luther is shown to have been of very slow growth, having lasted from 1512 to 1519.

[22] Alessandro Manzoni, a pupil of the Somascians, had been a revolutionary from his youth upwards. He deliberately wrote the words King, Emperor, and Pope without a capital letter. In Paris he came under the influence of Fauriel and Condorcet, who influenced the alteration of his artistic taste from that of the classical school to that of the romantic. His wife, who had been a Protestant, became converted to Catholicism, and was admitted into the Church in May, 1810. The example of his wife and the advice of two ecclesiastics determined Manzoni's own slow conversion from naturalistic religion to Catholicism. In 1811 the evolution of the conversion was complete. Guido Mazzoni emphatically states that it is purely mythical that Manzoni was converted suddenly by looking at an image of the Virgin, in one of the churches in Paris. His opinion is accepted by Giulio Salvadori, in his *Il rinnovamento d'Alessandro Manzoni e la sua riforma dell' arte* (Rome and Milan, 1910). It contains a good bibliography.

[23] For the conversion of Cardinal Newman see the note to Chapter IV.

[24] The description of his own conversion was given by Lutoslawskyi at the Geneva Congress in 1909. Cf. the Report of the Congress, op. cit. in Chapter I.

[25] The modern school of Catholic psychologists criticize all explanations of conversion and the phenomena of mysticism which are based on the unconscious. Cf. Pacheu, *L'Expérience mystique et l'activité subconsciente* (Paris, 1911). Cf. A. Gemelli, op. cit.

[26] Father Mainage, op. cit. See also " La conversione miracolosa di Alfonso Ratisbonne nel suo cinquantesimo anniversario ", in the *Civiltà Cattolica*, 22nd Feb., 1892.

[27] In my own religious experience, I myself remember having had, at long intervals, moments of this kind. I need relate only two of these experiences. The first occurred to me in 1908 at Assisi, in the *cortile* of the Capuchin Church. The other was in S. Maria Maggiore in Rome, in 1920, during a pontificial mass, at the moment when the choir were chanting the *descendit de Coelo*. Such experiences are inexpressible. But I may say that

of the experience of 1908 I find the following note written in my little diary: " Sadness; great mystery; the futility of human affairs." The second was characterized by a perception of a new meaning in the narrative passage of the *Credo*. At the time I had a rapid intuition of the fact of the Redemption; it was accompanied by a sensation of grandeur and by an ineffable solemnity. The association of ideas of the actual moment were the Holy Grail and Parsifal; after a few seconds the experience faded away, leaving no trace whatever, but a faint memory.

In point of fact, one of two things can happen : either the recollection is entirely lost, or can be recalled again, like any memory (as in my own case); or else it is retained in the mind by a deliberate effort of will and is insistently revived until the point at which the religious experience can be described and developed and criticized in rational terms. But none of this is what constitutes the actual conversion. Conversion, we repeat, is not a matter of theory, or a contemplation of states of consciousness; it is a question of conduct. The mutation of the individual necessitates his integral assent. The inspired may forget his own inspiration, but the convert can never be unmindful of his conversion, since he accepts his own experience.

[28] Many psychologists are of opinion that God works in the unconscious or in cœnæsthesia. This theory may be found either suggested or expounded in all the books and treatises dealing with mysticism.

[29] On this point it is worth while to insist on the fact that while the conversions to Roman Catholicism of young and of adult unbelievers, or of members of churches less organized, are numerous, conversions rapidly effected, or accompanied by exceptional phenomena, are of extreme rarity. At the Collegio Beda in Rome I learnt that of the fifteen English converts who were at the college in 1922, not one was converted suddenly; that none presented any extraordinary features, and that all of the conversions had been the outcome of a slow process. Monsignor Mann further declared that in England he had never seen unexpected and tumultuous conversions to Catholicism.

CHAPTER IV

[1] J. M. Baldwin, op. cit., *Dictionary of Philosophy and Psychology*, vol. ii, p. 356.

[2] Cf. Giuffrida-Ruggeri, *L'origine dell' uomo, nuove teorie e documenti* (Bologna, 1921). This book, which is a lucid résumé of the most modern knowledge on the subject, may serve

to orientate the unscientific reader. The author is a convinced and frequently polemical evolutionist. But while defending the zoological method and defining the limits of scientific research, he displays a commendable lucidity. Cf. in particular the preface to the book.

³ Those who are inclined to be scandalized by certain naturalistic similarities should be reminded that Goethe compared the emotions of an enamoured couple to the processes of chemical combination in his novel, which has an appropriately naturalistic title, *Die Wahlverwandtschaften* (Elective Affinities). Though the censorious might accuse the poet of materialism, no one would regard that as a reproach in a man of science, whose purpose is to study the significance of reality as a whole.

⁴ At the present time it is more prudent to indicate the relationship that exists between cosmic energy and vital energy, and between vital energy and psychic energy. It is generally maintained that vital energy does not come within the energetic cycle, any more than does psychic energy. This statement, however, while allowing full freedom of action to the materialists, who deny the existence of any form of energy other than physicochemical, does not absolutely shut the door on any other theoretical interpretation. In spite of the controversial nature and the obscurity of the conception of psychic energy, it has been adopted by numerous psychologists. It is here sufficient to mention Alfred Lehmann, and his *Psychodynamik*. But the reader will have understood the sense in which we allude to it.

On the subject of Psychic Energy see Theodor Lipps, *Leitfaden der Psychologie* (3rd edition, Leipzig, 1909). A totally different view of psychic energy is to be found in W. Ostwald's book, *Die Energie* (1908). The French translation, here quoted, is *L'Energie* (Paris, 1910). See also *Esquisse d'une philosophie des sciences* (Paris, 1911). A somewhat more recent psychological publication on the subject of Energetics is the *Psychologia energetica* of Rodriquez Etchart (Buenos Aires, 1913).

⁵ Pierre Janet, " La tension psychologique et ses oscillations " in the *Journal de psych. normal et path.* (May and June, 1915). Cf. also " Les oscillations de l'activité mentale ", ibid., Jan., 1920.

⁶ The *Bewusstseinslage* has been the subject of many treatises and studies, but its nature still remains very obscure. According to some authorities, its derivation is to be traced back to individual tendencies. It is here opportune to recall the Freudian theory of the *Ich-Komplex*, or ego-complex, which Freud regards as constituting the unity of the psychic personality.

⁷ Sigmund Freud, *Über Psychoanalyse* (Vienna and Leipzig, 1922). Cf. Lecture III, where the author deals with the subject of complexes. See further Otto Selz, *Über die Gesetze des geordneten*

Denkverlaufs (Stuttgart, 1913) ; also an article by the same writer, on the " Komplextheorie und Konstellationstheorie ", in the *Zeitschrift für Psychologie,* vol. lxxxiii.

[8] This monistic conception is clearly discoverable in art. Goethe, in *Faust,* expresses it thus :—

> " Zwar ist's mit der Gedankenfabrik
> Wie mit einem Webermeisterstück,
> Wo ein Tritt tausend Fäden regt,
> Die Schifflein herüber, hinüber schiessen,
> Die Fäden ungesehen fliessen.
> Ein Schlag tausend Verbindungen schlägt."

" The fabric of thought is even as the work of weaver's loom : by a single movement of the treadle a thousand threads are set in motion. The shuttle flies, the unseen threads run, and at a single stroke a thousand connections are interwoven."

[9] W. Wundt, *Gründzüge der physiologischen Psychologie,* sixth edition (Leipzig, 1911), vol. iii. English translation : *Principles of Physiological Psychology* (London, 1904).

[10] There is an immense modern literature on the subject of the physiological basis of the affective life, and more particularly of the sympathetic and endocrine systems. An excellent bibliography—which also includes works on pathology—may be found in a recent work by Vito Maria Buscaino : *Biologia della vita emotiva* (Bologna, 1922).

[11] Cf. Sante De Sanctis, *Psychologie des Traumes,* op. cit.

[12] Hermann Ronge, the hero described by Jœrgensen in *Dal pelago alla riva,* already mentioned.

[13] St. John of the Cross, *Obras del venerable Padre Fray Juan de la Cruz,* Madrid, 1649, and Seville, 1703. English translation : *The Complete Works of St. John of the Cross ;* translated from the original Spanish by D. Lewis ; edited by the Oblate Fathers of St. Charles, with a Preface by Cardinal Wiseman (London, 1864). A good modern Spanish edition is that edited by Marcelino Menéndez y Pelayo in 3 vols. (Toledo, 1912). The Italian edition here referred to is : *Le Opere complete di S. Giovanni della Croce,* translated by P. F. Marco di S. Francesco, preceded by a Foreword by P. Berthier (Como, 1859).

[14] The Rev. R. A. Knox, *A Spiritual Aeneid,* which was published in 1918, is quoted by Father Mainage, op. cit.

[15] This testimony is by Georges Dumesnil in Father Mainage's *Nos Convertis,* op. cit.

[16] Much has already been written on the subject of Giovanni Papini's conversion. It has been doubted by some, while others firmly believe in the change that has taken place in him. I base my own opinion on the accounts given by the author's friends,

such as Vanni and Moscardelli, and also by what he has written himself. His letter to Signor Mazzucconi appears to me to be explicit. Even more explicit is Moscardelli, who has been the confidant of the author of the *Storia di Cristo*. Papini's case may be regarded rather as a conversion than either a ' return ' or a ' recognition ', since if one is to believe in the existence of Papini's previous Christianity at all, it cannot be said that he expressed such faith in his life. His conversion influenced his activity and life ; and it is on this account a true conversion. But it may be asked : Of what type was Papini's conversion ? Surely the progressive. His regeneration was already apparent in his book *Un uomo finito*, published in 1912.

N. Moscardelli, who has described Papini's preparation for conversion—the profounder depths of the mutational process— at the same time indicates and confirms the theory of conversion which I have outlined in the present work. From Moscardelli's own article on Giovanni Papini, in the *Tempo* of 2nd May, 1921, I quote the following words : " . . . Even while he was demolishing, vituperating, and blaspheming one felt that all the destruction, vituperation, and blasphemy filled his mouth only, but not his heart. One felt that so open and candid a detestation was purely on the surface, and that the depth of his soul only awaited the touch of a powerful hand to become revealed. He had a great need of love, because only those who are rich in love have need of love. But what was he to love ? We can feign to be God, because the flesh is always ready to agree to such betrayals, but the spirit will not drink of such water. One may destroy what exists, but the soul impassioned of love will not content itself with overthrow, because love seeks to create. One may retire to ruminate upon the failure of the attack, counting the wounded, and wishing the same fate of those still fighting. But the soul possessed by love cannot shut itself up in itself, just as a fire cannot be covered without being extinguished. Only death, or a new life, can give this peace. For those who are worthy of it, this is precisely the time in which this new life is born."

[17] There is an accurate bibliography of Cardinal Newman, among other modern writers on religious subjects, in Giuseppe Prezzolini's *Il Cattolicismo rosso* (Naples, 1908). On Newman see also the writings of H. Brémond, and of Ernest Dimnet, and the introduction to the Italian translation of Newman's *Grammar of Assent* (*Fede e Ragione*) by Battaini, who also gives a brief biography of the famous Cardinal (Turin, 1907). The English edition was published in London in 1889. Cf. in particular the five chapters of the first part. The reader should not fail to read J. H. Newman's *Apologia pro vita sua* (London, 1913).

[18] The facts concerning Pusey and Newman I have taken from

many sources. See H. S. Liddon's *Life of Edward Bouverie Pusey* (London, 4 vols., 1893-4). Cf. particularly Henri Brémond's *L'inquiétude religieuse, Aubes et lendemains de conversion* (2nd edition, Paris, 1903). This work was crowned by the French Academy. The author is extremely well informed. He was in England and knew Pusey and the Oxford religious movement. He is an enthusiastic admirer of Cardinal Newman.

[19] On the subject of Conviction, see J. Jastrow, *The Psychology of Conviction, A Study of Belief and Attitudes* (Boston, 1918). Cf. also Eugenio Rignano, *Psicologia del ragionamento* (Milan, 1921) [E. T. *The Psychology of Reasoning* in the " International Library of Psychology, Philosophy, and Scientific Method", 1923.] F. Mentrè, *Espèces et variétés d'intelligence, Eléments de Noologie* (Paris, 1920). The author endeavours to explain the differences of opinions and the varieties of doctrines of man, according to the various types of psychical make-up.

[20] It must be clearly understood that my intention here is to give a simple scheme. It is not altogether devoid of significance that even the religious teachers to-day make appeal to psychological and scientific theories. Cf. Gerhard Füllkrug, *Zur Seelenkunde der weiblichen Jugend, Die Neugeburt des Ich* (Schwerin a/M., 1913), second edition.

[21] La Fontaine was an upright, ingenuous, frank soul, as André Hallays says in his articles, " Jean de la Fontaine", in the *Revue des Deux Mondes*, 1921. He offered very little resistance to the call of ' grace ' and readily admitted the impropriety of his *Contes* at the Abbé Poucet's instigation. On 13th January, 1693, La Fontaine received the Viaticum, two years before his death. During his two last years, he maintained his conversion, it would seem, with strength and constancy. But it was said that he had become greatly enfeebled mentally by his illness, though this is denied by some of his biographers. It is, indeed, certain that after his conversion the poet's tastes and habits were unchanged, and that he continued to write poetry and fables. He died on 13th April, 1695, " avec une constance admirable et toute chrétienne", as we are told by Charles Perrault. When his body was laid out for burial, he was discovered to be wearing a hair-shirt. Georges Izambard speaks of the conversion of La Fontaine in connection with the occasion of the tercentenary of the poet. This writer says explicitly that during the two years which followed La Fontaine's conversion, brought about by the famous Abbé Poucet, " he was nothing but a poor old madman, the prey of fits of delirous mysticism." But this appears to be a hasty conclusion.

[22] Cf. an article by Müller-Freienfels in the *Zeitschs. für Psychol.*, etc., 1914.

²³ Th. Ribot, *Problèmes de psychologie affective* (Paris, 1910). The author gives a summary of his ideas on the affective states and upon cœnæsthesia, the tendencies, and the instincts. See also Ribot's *La vie inconsciente et les mouvements* (Paris, 1914). In this work the author maintains that the entire psychic life is dominated by motor activity, existing in the unconscious and becoming united to the affect in the state of consciousness.

²⁴ On the theory of *Verschiebung*, or displacement, or transposition, or transference, in addition to the works of Freud, of which mention has already been made, cf. also Assagioli, Levi-Bianchini, Weiss, etc.

²⁵ The transference and substitution of tendencies, from the primordial to the highest and most complex, is a biological concept much exploited by evolutionists. Cf. Rignano, *The Psychology of Reasoning*, op. cit., and a critique of Sante De Sanctis in the *Rivista di Psicologia*, by G. C. Ferrari and G. Tarozzi, July and September, 1921.

²⁶ This transposition is clearly seen in St. John of the Cross, *Salita del Carmelo*, chap. xv, p. 110, of the Italian edition, op. cit. The Saint, in the *Notte Oscura*, Book I, chap. xi, and elsewhere, gives an explanation of the subject of transference or transposition, for instance, when he comments on his own phrase : " From the madness of burning love, wherefrom I languished."

²⁷ The majority of psychiatric text-books omit to mention ' transitivism ' specifically. An exception, however, is Martin Reichardt, who alludes to it in the 2nd edition of his *Allgemeine und spezielle Psychiatrie*, etc. (Jena, 1918), p. 67. This author writes that it is a case of transitivism, when, for instance, the mental patient believes that those of his *entourage* are mentally affected. The writer who deals most exhaustively with this subject is E. Bleuler, cf. *Lehrbuch der Psychiatrie* (Berlin, 1906), English translation, *Textbook of Psychiatry* (New York and London, 1923). On p. 34 of the English edition he observes that the influence of affectivity on thought and action is reinforced by its *tendency to spread*. In point of time the affects usually outlast the corresponding intellectual phenomena, and easily ' radiate ' to other psychic experiences which are associated in some way with the idea in question. Thus we love the place where we have experienced something beautiful, but hate the innocent bearer of bad news. Love may be ' transferred ' from one person to another bearing some analogy to the first, or to some object such as a letter. Even in normal conditions the transferred affect may detach itself from the original idea so that this becomes indifferent, while the second idea carries the affect which does not properly belong to it. (Displacement of the affect.)

In the chapter on Disturbances of the Personality, p. 138, et seq., Bleuler describes the mechanism of ' transitivism ', by which the personality may become dissociated in such a way that part of the patient's experiences become separated from him and attributed to some other person. For instance, a patient sees a terrifying face and screams, but thinks it is the face that has screamed. In dreams we habitually transfer the emotions we ourselves feel to some other person. In dementia præcox this transitivism is a most common sympton. Patients are persuaded that the voices which they hear must necessarily be heard in the same way by others. They frequently attribute their own actions to other persons ; for example, when they read something, it is others who have done so, or their thoughts are thought by others. Indeed, among the schizophrenes there is a distinct dissociation of the affect from the representative group. The Freudians say that the psychic load is withdrawn from the objects of the external world and transported elsewhere.

It must be clearly emphasized that the morbidness does not lie in the dissociation itself—which is a normal phenomenon—but in the modes of dissociation and in the material which is dissociated. It is a common characteristic among the insane, for example, to separate words from the conception they express, and to transfer them to other ideas.

[28] For the psychiatric conception of ' Introjection ', the reader is referred to the interesting work of S. Ferenczi, *Introjektion und Übertragung ; eine psycho-analytische Studie* (Vienna and Leipzig, 1910).

[29] I. Petrone, *Ascetica* (Naples, 1918). To be quite accurate, in another passage, i.e. in chapter xviii, Petrone recognizes that the passions should not be *entirely* suppressed.

[30] B. Croce, *Filosofia della pratica* (Bari, 1909). [E. T., *Philosophy of the Practical* (London, 1913).]

CHAPTER V

[1] Havelock Ellis, *The Evolution of Modesty*, vol. i of *Studies in the Psychology of Sex* (Philadelphia, 1902). The French edition is here quoted : *La pudeur*, p. 382. The literature on the biological aspect of the sexual instinct is exceedingly voluminous, and there is no necessity to quote it. The works of Havelock Ellis in general, and especially the volume on *The Analysis of the Sexual Impulse*, vol. iii of *Studies in the Psychology of Sex* (Philadelphia, 1903), French edition : *L'Impulsion Sexuelle* (Paris, 1911), will serve

to orientate the reader, cf. chapter i. Of still more importance are the works of Albert Moll, and particularly his *Handbuch des Sexualwissenschaften* (Leipzig, 1912). It contains a large bibliography. The more recent researches of Steinach are also noteworthy.

² Ivan Bloch, *Das Sexualleben* (English translation, *The Sexual Life of our Time*). Italian translation by Carrara (Turin, 1910), cf. chap. vi, " L'Idealismo dell' Amore." Of interest also is L. Feuerbach's *Il culto di Maria*, quoted by Bloch in chapter v.

³ *Lo spirito di San Francesco ed il Terz'ordine*, a work by Dr. Dietrich von Hildebrand, Italian translation by Giulia Citterio Glas (Munich, 1921).

⁴ Antonio Fogazzaro, *Discorsi* (Milan, 1912), cf. the lecture on " La Figura di Antonio Rosmini ".

⁵ Freud, *Vorlesungen zur Einführung in die Psycho-analyse* (Vienna, 1918). (English translation, *Introductory Lectures on Psycho-analysis*, London, 1922). Cf. Part III.

⁶ A. Paolucci, *A spiritu fornicationis*, 1920 (issued for private circulation only).

⁷ Johannes Jœrgensen, *Dal Pelago alla riva*, op. cit. As is well known, this author is a convert from the positivist school of Brandes to Catholicism. His conversion took place in 1896.

⁸ Comte de Montalambert, *Historie de Sainte Elisabeth de Hongrie, duchesse de Thuringie*, in 2 vols, 27th edition (Paris, 1920), a documented historical biography.

⁹ St. François de Sales. *Introduction à la vie devote* ; texte integral d'après l'édition de 1619, Nelson's edition (Paris undated).

¹⁰ Harnack, *Der ' Eros ' in der alten Arist. Literatur* (Berlin, 1918).

¹¹ *Fioretti di San Francesco*, op. cit., p. 109.

¹² The works of St. John the Cross, op. cit., cf. the *Salita del Carmelo*, Book I, chapter ii.

¹³ On this subject see : Henry Joly's *Sainte Thérèse* (13th edition, Paris, 1919), and Cazal's *Sainte Thérèse* (Paris, 1921). From the latter the quotation from Saint Gertrude is taken.

¹⁴ *Fioretti*, op. cit.

¹⁵ H. Joly, op. cit., cf. p. 224.

¹⁶ J. Jœrgensen, *Sainte Catherine de Sienne* (Paris, 1919).

¹⁷ R. Maulde de La Clavière, *Vie de St. Gaëtan* (2nd edition, Paris, 1905). There is also an Italian translation of this work by A. Castaldo, with a preface by Giulio Salvadori (Rome, 1911).

¹⁸ Bl. Cardinal Bellarmine, *De ascensione mentis in Deum per scalas rerum creatarum* (Paris, 1606) ; quoted on p. 30 of La Clavière, op. cit.

¹⁹ It is related in the *Fioretti* that Brother Corrado, having said his prayers, there appeared to him the Queen of Heaven, with

her Child in her arms, amid a great splendour of light ; and that, coming near to the monk, she placed the infant in his arms ; and that the friar embraced Him, and held Him close, and kissed Him, and was dissolved in divine love, with inexpressible consolation.

On the subject of the visions of St. Gaetan, it must be added that La Clavière (op. cit.) admits on p. 39 that in the year 1517 to 1518, the saint " vivait dans un état d'éxaltation qui diminuait en lui le sens du réel."

[20] Benedetto Croce, *Filosofia della pratica*, op. cit., English translation, *Philosophy of the Practical*.

[21] Paulhan, *Les transformations sociales des sentiments* (Paris, 1920). The individual is always incompletely unified. Society presents still further incoherencies ; these cases are the outcome of imperfect adjustments to imperfect systems. Individual and social pathology and the maladjustments of social conditions, therefore, always contain the latent germs of asystemization, or anarchy. Spiritualization is a co-ordination of tendencies and of ideas which is superior to the synthetic unity of the organic needs and appetites. Idealization, on the other hand, consists in the purification, or sublimation, of these tendencies. At times idealization approaches spiritualization, at other times it is the opposite. Socialization is the outcome of social solidarity.

In Part II of *Les transformations*, Paulhan alludes to the spiritualization and the socialization of the sexual impulse. Love is the result of a spiritualization—always incomplete—of the sexual instinct. On pages 221 to 227 he maintains that mysticism is derived from love.

[22] On the subject of ' censoring ', as on the subject of sublimation, and generally on what happens to unconscious desires when unveiled, the reader may consult Sigmund Freud, *Über Psychoanalyse* (Vienna and Leipzig, 1922), and idem, *Vorlesungen zur Einführung*, etc., op. cit., Lecture XXII. The theories of Freud on the subject are that the sexual instincts (*Sexuelle Triebregungen*) are extraordinarily plastic and that it is perfectly possible, therefore, for one to become substituted for another. It is also possible for one of these to acquire the intensity proper to another. Hence, when reality necessitates the renunciation of one impulse, another may be invested with its affect, and give full compensation for the satisfaction denied to the other. These impulses act like a network of intercommunicating canals, filled with fluid, and this in spite of their subjection to the primacy of the genitalia (the *Genitalprimat*). Besides this, the partial instincts of sexuality, like the sexual tendency (or *Sexualstrebung*) which is composed of all these, possess the faculty of being readily

able to alter their objective (*Objekt*) or of exchanging that objective for another, which is more easily obtained. This displacement and disposition (or *Bereitwilligkeit*) to accept a surrogate must prove a powerful preventive agent against the pathogenic results of frustration (*Versagung*). Among these processes which protect the subject against disorders arising out of *Versagung*, one has assumed a special cultural importance. It consists in this : that the sexual tendency (or *Sexualstrebung*), when deflected from its goal (*Ziel*), either of a partial pleasure (*Partiallust*) or that of procreation, takes up a new aim which is in genetic nexus with the one abandoned. But the new aim is no longer sexual, and may be said to be social. We call this process sublimation, in accordance with the general valuation, which places the aims of society higher than sexual aims, which are ultimately selfish (*selbstsüchtig*). Sublimation, according to Freud, is, indeed, nothing but a special case of the leaning (*Anlehnung*) of sexual tendencies (*Sexualstrebungen*) upon non-sexual tendencies. In *Über Psychoanalyse*, op. cit., Freud deals in Lecture V with the censor and with sublimation.

See also R. Assagioli, on the conception of sublimation, in " Trasformazioni e sublimazione delle energie sessuali ", in the *Rivista di Psic. applicata*, vii, 1911. For a criticism of sublimation in the sense of Freud see Rudolf Allers, " Psychologie des Geschlechtslebens," in Kafka's *Handbuch*, op. cit., vol. iii. The writer admits that sexuality plays a part in religious experience, but denies that it is the whole of religious emotion. And of this all are convinced, as I myself have already stated, in the text.

²³ Smith Ely Jelliffe, *The Technique of Psycho-analysis*, op. cit., p. 42.

²⁴ On this point, and in connection with Jung, the reader is referred to the *Bericht über die Fortschritte der Psychoanalyse*, op. cit. Cf. chapter i. See also C. G. Jung, *Wandlungen und Symbole der Libido* (Leipzig and Vienna, 1912) (English translation *The Psychology of the Unconscious*, New York, 1916, and London, 1921). The author defines his own theoretical conception of the libido, which he places above its purely sexual signification, bringing it back again to its interpretation in the classical or Ciceronian sense, as meaning passionate desire in general. The views of Jung also deserve a full discussion, in regard to their application to psycho-pathology.

I have always thought that the furious endeavour to get down to the origins of psycho-pathological phenomena led fatally towards uniformity. It is to be observed that recent psycho-pathologists, such as Jaspers, recognize two different methods in

mental pathology : the *causal* and the *psycho-genetic*. This seems
to be an entirely logical conception, though I cannot accept it
without reserves. Working backwards towards origins, one
certainly comes to the libido, as conceived by Jung. This, however, is not sufficient to account for all the phenomena of psychopathology, since certain remote origins are common to the most
divergent phenomena. For these reasons I hold that the conception of psychic ' connections ' should be substituted for that
of psycho-genesis. Interconnections and interferences are more
important than the ultimate origin.

[25] Cf. S. Freud's *Vorlesungen*, op. cit.

[26] Rudolph Eucken, *Die Lebensanschauungen der grossen
Denker : Eine Entwickelungsgeschichte des Lebensproblems der
Menschheit von Plato bis zur Gegenwart* (Leipzig, 1902). English
translation : *The Problem of Human life as viewed by Great
Thinkers from Plato to the Present Time* (London, 1909). *La
visione della vita nei grandi pensatori*, Italian translation by
P. Martinetti (Turin, 1909), p. 218.

[27] Cf. L. Bertrand, *St. Augustin*, op. cit., p. 450 et seq. But this
observation does not exclude the view that St. Augustine had
succeeded in accomplishing the sublimation of the libido. This
is what Werner Achelis has endeavoured to show in *Die Deutung
Augustins Bischof von Hippo. Analyse seines geistigen Schaffens
auf Grund seiner erotischen Struktur* (Trier, 1921). This interesting
book throws a light on the importance of sublimated,
or repressed, sexuality for the activity of the religious
soul. The writer shows that St. Augustine, by his conversion, had
achieved the sublimation of his eroticism. He maintains, however,
that there remained in him a certain residue of his eroticism, which
was unsublimated, and that this manifested itself in phenomena
of repressions and neuroses. The book is ambitious in its aims
and deals with many—indeed, too many—subjects. For that
reason, it interests us only in parts.

[28] Giovanni Papini, *Storia di Cristo* (Florence, 1921). (English
translation : *The Life of Christ*, 1923.)

[29] The criticisms of a psychological order by Padre Barbèra
on my lecture on Conversion applied specifically to this point.
On the subject of sublimation he objected that the theory of
Freud was " highly dangerous ". It is, however, certain that he
has not fully understood the process of sublimation, since he
believes it to be a completely unknowable process. I am keenly
interested in the psychology of Freud, but not at all in his
philosophical theories. The process of sublimation which has, and
has always had, its roots in biology, can certainly evolve without
volition and without consciousness. But it is equally true that at
a certain stage of its development it can become not only conscious

but emphatically volitional. In fact, true sublimation is accomplished with effort and with sacrifice. The writer in his critique discriminates between that emotion of delight, which accompanies and completes the accomplished work, and the emotion of desire, an impulse more or less sensitive, which is unconscious; and he declares that will is often confounded with feeling, whereas the former is self-conscious and the latter is blind. This distinction is right, but I do not see how it can serve as the basis of a critique of my lecture.

[30] Ribot, *La Logique des sentiments* (Paris, 1905). Cf. in particular, p. 175 et seq.

[31] *La Bienheureuse Marguerite-Marie* (*1647–1690*), by Monsignor Deminuid (Paris, 1912). *La Beata Margherita Maria Alacoque*, Italian edition translated from the French (Rome, 1912).

[32] Languet, quoted by Deminuid, op. cit.

[33] Freud, *Vorlesungen*, op. cit., Lecture XXII, on the Etiology of General Neuroses, says that neuroses may arise when there is no possibility of satisfying the libido, and 'privation' (*Versagung*) occurs; and that the neurotic symptoms are a substitution for the satisfaction (*Befriedigung*) that is denied. Naturally, not every *Versagung* results in a neurosis, but in all neurotics a *Versagung* can be demonstrated. The privation is rarely complete and absolute. To be pathogenic it must strike at that mode of satisfaction which the whole personality demands, and of which alone it is capable. But there are usually a number of ways of enduring the lack of satisfaction of the libido without neurotic ailments. There assuredly are men who are capable of enduring this privation without injury; they are not happy, they experience longings (*Sehnsucht*), but they do not become ill.

[34] The convert Paul Claudel declared that "what prevents people from becoming religious is the repugnance they feel at relinquishing pleasurable things". De Borden writes: "To all those who would be converted I say that if they feel the courage, they should give themselves up to God without delay; they should throw themselves into Him as one throws oneself into the sea to swim; and God will take care of them and will remove from them every internal conflict," etc. Agostino Fattori refers to this in his *Confessione*, in a letter to Vincenzo Cento. Cf. *Bylichnis*, March, 1920. But the most eloquent example is that of Durtal, in Huysmans's *En Route*.

[35] St. John of the Cross, op. cit., chap. iv.

[36] St. Gregory recalls the powerful temptation of the flesh in the case of St. Benedict and how the saint finally overcame it by throwing himself into thorns. The story of Benedict is well

known. He fled from Rome in his boyhood, at the age of about twenty, abandoning the aristocratic girl whom he loved (a member, perhaps, of the Merula family) and by whom he was deeply loved in return. He took up his abode in the solitude of Subiaco, and there realized that sublimation which he desired, filled with the example of the legends of the anchorites of Egypt and of Palestine brought to Rome by the Bishop Athanasius.

[37] On these questions the reader is referred to L. Löwenfeld, *Über die sexuelle Konstitution und andere Sexualprobleme* (Wiesbaden, 1911).

[38] As is well known, the internal secretions of the sexual glands are not the work of the entire testicle or the entire ovary, but of the specialized cells, called interstitial (or the " gland of puberescence ", according to Steinach) in both the male and the female. There appears to be no doubt of this specialization in the case of mammals. The recent objections to this theory refer to other animal species. In mammals the interstitial cells function as glands of internal secretion, while the ovary and the testicle function as generative glands. The feminization of a castrated male may be produced by the secretions of an ovary grafted in him, and the masculization of a female may be obtained by a corresponding testicular graft. Steinach has, thereby, experimentally produced sex, even as regards the sexual characteristics. In the cases in which Steinach grafted both an ovary and testicles upon a castrated animal, he produced a hermaphrodite. There are acceleratory and retardatory hormones of metabolism, or disassimilative and assimilative (Biedl), or catabolic and anabolic. According to Falta. the glands of the interstitial cells are retardatory or anabolic, whilst the generative glands belong to the catabolic group and are disassimilative or accelerative. In the pre-menstrual period all the vital processes are augmented.

To obtain a clear idea of the glands of internal secretion, cf: A. Weil, *Die innere Sekretion, Eine Einführung f. Studierende u. Aerzte* (Berlin, 1921). This volume clearly indicates the connection between the sexual life and the internal secretions, according to the recent views, not only of Biedl and Pende, but also of Tandler, Steinach, Lichtenstern, Mühsam, etc. Cf. also L. R. Müller, *Das vegetative Nervensystem*, in collaboration with Dahl, Glaser, Greving, Zierl, etc. (Berlin, 1920) ; and also Lerebouillet, Hanvier, Guillaume, and Carrion, *Sympathique et glandes endocrines* (Paris, 1921). This book is well illustrated and places the reader conveniently *au courant* with the main arguments. The celebrated work of Falta has been translated into English (*Endocrine Diseases*, 1923), and Italian (*Le Malattie delle glandole sanguigne*, Milan, 1914). As this discussion has become fashionable, the bibliography of the subject has grown extensively in all languages during the last two years. But additional citations are not needed.

[39] In recent times a great number of authors have tried to trace a connection between the internal secretions of the endocrine glands and the moral states. Among Italians the chief authority is Nicola Pende, who has published a résumé of his views : " Endocrinologia e Psicologia," in *Quaderni di Psichiatria* (Genoa, 1921).

[40] Carlo Ceni, *Cervello e funzioni materne. Saggio di Fisiologia e Psicologia comparata*, 2 vols. (Turin and Genoa, 1922).

CHAPTER VI

[1] St. Theresa (de Cepeda) of Jesus. *Cartas de Santa Teresa de Jesus*, con notas de Senor Don J. de Palafox y Mendoza, Madrid and Saragosa, 1671 (English translation : *The Letters of St. Theresa*, translated by the Benedictines of Stanbrook, with a Preface by Cardinal Gasquet, London, 1919-23).

The edition cited in the text is the Italian version : *Lettere della Santa Madre Teresa di Gesù*, with the annotations of Monsignore Gio. di Palafox y Mendoza, translated into the Italian by Carlo Sigismondo Capece (Venice, 1690).

Las Obras de la Santa Madre Teresa de Jesus. De nuevo corregido, with a preface by L. Ponce de Leon, (Lisbon, Antonio Alvarez, 1616) [English translation, London, 1913-19]. The Italian edition here quoted is *Opere spirituale della Santa Madre Teresa di Gesù* (Venice, 1650).

[2] James, *Varieties of Religious Experience*, op. cit.

[3] The edition quoted is the Italian version : *L'Ornamento delle nozze spirituale* of Jan van Ruysbroeck, translated into Italian, with an introduction by D. Giuliotti (Carabba, 1916). See also the French edition, *Oeuvres de Ruysbroeck, L'Admirable*, translated from the Flemish by the Benedictines of St. Paul de Wisques, 3rd edition revised and corrected (Brussels, 1919). [English translation, *The Adornment of the Spiritual Marriage, the Book of Truth and the Sparkling Stone*, translated by C. A. Wynschenk, Dom., London, 1916.]

[4] Father Bernard Christhien D'Andermatt, op. cit.

[5] G. Truc, " Les états mystiques négatifs", in *Revue Philosophique* (1912, p. 610).

[6] M. de Montmorand, *Psychologie des Mystiques* (Paris, 1920), in which the author speaks of the oscillations of the mental levels of mystics ; see chapter ii. He deals with the theological explanation (the doctrines of purgation and purification, active or passive), to which is opposed the theory of Murisier and

Godfernaux, which is based on the variations of organic consciousness, or cœnæsthesia.

[7] S. De Sanctis, " Les enfants dysthymiques," in *Encephale* (Paris, 1922) : and " I fanciulli distimici " in *Infanzia anormale* (Milan, 1921).

[8] Ségond, *La Prière* (Paris, 1911). See also the *Raccolta delle Conferenze sulla Preghiera fatte presso il Circolo di studi religiosi in Roma*, conference held in 1922 (about to be published).

[9] Dante alludes to Poverty at length, in connection with St. Francis.

> . . . *per tal donna [poverty] giovinetto in guerra*
> *Del padre corse, a cui, com' alla morte,*
> *La porta del piacer nessun disserra.*
> *E dinanzi alla sua spirital Corte*
> *Et coram patre le si fece unito ;*
> *Poscia di dì in dì l'amò più forte.*
> *Questa, privata del primo marito [Christ]*
> *Mille e cent' anni e più dispetta e scura*
> *Fino a costui si stette senza invito.*
>
> .   .   .   .
>
> *Francesco e Povertà per questi amanti*
> *Prendi oramai nel mio parlar diffuso.*
>
> (*Parad.* XI, 58–75.)

" For such lady's sake, a youth, he ran upon his father's enmity, that to her, as to death, none unlocks the gate of pleasure ; and in presence of his spiritual court *et coram patre* he became united to her ; afterward from day to day he loved her more strongly. She, bereaved of her first husband (Christ), eleven hundred years and more despised and obscure, until his time remained without wooing ; . . . Take now in my diffuse speech Francis and Poverty for these lovers."

This clearly shows the association of love and poverty and the mystic union between Poverty and St. Francis in the mind of the poet as in Giotto's.

[10] Wundt, *Principles of Physiological Psychology*, op. cit., vol. iii.

[11] Benedetto Croce, *Breviario di Estetica* (Bari, 1920–4). English translation : *The Essence of Aesthetic* (London, 1921).

[12] The Essays and Aphorisms of Otto Weininger, *Über die letzten Dinge, mit einem biographischen Vorwort von M. Rappaport* (Vienna and Leipzig, 1904). Italian translation, *Intorno alle cose supreme* (Turin, 1914), p. 53.

[13] Professor Flournoy translated the German term *Einfühlung* by the French word *Intropathie*. For an account of *Einfühlung* the reader should consult Th. Lipps's *Leitfaden der Psychologie*, 3rd edition (Leipzig, 1909). See also Benedetto Croce, *Estetica*

come scienza dell' espressione e linguistica generale (3rd edition, Bari, 1909). The author herein expounds his famous theory of aesthetics, and gives an historical account of other theories. He alludes to the conception of *Einfühlung* in chapter xviii of the second part.

[14] N. Turchi, *Storia delle religioni* (Turin, 1912). Second edition published in 1922. This book has an admirable bibliography. Cf. also *History of Religions* by George Foot Moore (London, 2 vols, 1914-20) on the same subject, which has been translated into Italian by Professor Lapiana. (*Storia delle Religione*, Bari, 1922.) In two volumes.

[15] Cf. the translation of the Blessed Angela of Foligno's book, *Il Libro delle mirabili visioni e consolazioni*, etc. (Florence, 1922). There is also the celebrated work on the Blessed Angela of Foligno by E. Hello. The allusions to her by Huysmans, in his *En Route*, are well known.

[16] The ideas of Gentile on the subject of the relationship between idealistic philosophy and religion have been fully elaborated in his various publications. I must content myself by referring here to his *Il modernismo e i rapporti tra religione e filosofia*, op. cit., chapter i, and to his *Discorsi di religione* (Florence, 1920). A conscientious but critical account of the actualistic idealism of Giovanni Gentile may be found in a volume of Emilio Chiocchetti's *La filosofia di G. Gentile* (Milan, 1922). Read chapter vi. It would not appear that Gentile's conception of auto-conscious reality entirely corresponds to identification. Gentile considers that auto-consciousness is subjective, but that the subject is such inasmuch as it is objective to itself. In fact, it is a case of auto-objectivation. However, both in Gentile's philosophic views and in those of his disciples, identificatory conceptions are to be found which leave no doubts. Gentile declares that the divine is the absolute negation of the subject; that in religion the subject is forgotten, submerged, annulled, dissolved in the object, and so forth. It seems, however, that even for these idealists, the annulment that occurs is transitory, *sui generis*: and, according to Gentile himself, the position of the object is really determined in the presence of the subject.

[17] The reader is referred to the teachings of St. Paul and to the doctrines of the Gnostics. See the work of E. Bonajuti, *Lo Gnosticismo* (Rome, 1907). See p. 27 et seq.

[18] See, for an account of the Third Order of St. Francis, Dr. Dietrich von Hildebrand, op. cit., chapter v, note 3.

[19] Professor Karl Jaspers, *Psychologie der Weltanschauungen* (Berlin, 1919). See in *Psychosen*, " Der Absolute Nihilismus," p. 265.

[20] Cf. the text-books on mental diseases, generally, and, in particular, L. Dugas and F. Moutier, *La dépersonalisation* (Paris, 1911), with a bibliography. This volume should serve to give a fairly complete description of the particular affective theory held by French psychopathologists, as regards the phenomena of dissociation of the personality.

[21] See Phaneg's " Étude sur l'envoûtement ", a paper read before the Société d'études psychiques de Nancy, published in *Echo du Merveilleux*, 1906. *L'envoûtement* was scientifically explained, but Jules Grasset in *L'occultisme : hier et aujourd'hui* (Paris, 1907), p. 363, says in a note that the subject of this argument is still not ripe for scientific discussion. Projection may be said to be the basis of magic performances. Cf. A. Sacchi, *Istituzoni di scienza occulta* (Turin, 1906), the work of a convinced believer in magic.

CHAPTER VII

[1] The literature of psychiatry dealing with religious subjects, mysticism, holiness, prophecy—other than genius, with which we are not here concerned—is extremely voluminous. I would limit myself to mentioning Dr. Wilhelm Hirsch, *Religion und Civilisation vom Standpunkte des Psychiaters* (Munich, 1910), reviewed in the *Archiv. für die ges. Psychol.* (xxix, parts 3 and 4, 1913). Apparently Hirsch regards every Biblical personage as afflicted with *manie de grandeur*. The author considers the Bible literally in its accounts and in its various figures. Abraham, according to the author, was a student of the natural sciences, a mathematician and an astronomer, who was obliged to leave his native land for Canaan, on account of his maniacal monotheistic ideas. The sacrifice of Isaac is, for Hirsch, a proof of Abraham's insanity. All the writings of the prophets, from Isaiah and Jeremiah down to Malachi, were mere expressions of the confusion and disconnection of their diseased brains. Jesus gave indications of delusions of grandeur (by talking of a divine origin, of his own divinity, and of his kingdom). In dealing with the history of Christianity the author makes it responsible for all the evils perpetrated in its name.

As so frequently occurs, this book is based on a cardinal psychiatric error regarding the conception of insanity. Why is it the author fails to explain how Jeremiah—a visionary—was none the less recognized as a strong personality in the history of Israel ?

In Italy the attention of psychologists has been directed with some insistence to the investigations into the connection between religion and insanity by Dr. Portigliotti, to which reference will be made later.

² Otto Meyerhof, *Beiträge zur psychologischen Theorie der Geistesstörungen* (Göttingen, 1910), cf. p. 77.

³ Charles Blondel, *La conscience morbide* (Paris, 1914). [A short account of the author's theory will be found in *Psyche*, vol. vi, London, 1926.] This is an interesting book on account of its fundamental conception, to which reference has been made in the text. The ' pure psychologist ' in us is composed of the homogeneous mass of our organic impressions, incapable of being conceptualized themselves or of becoming rational and logical. Modifications of cœnæsthesia may occur without the mental state being thereby altered (tabes). On the other hand, consciousness becomes morbid when the ' pouring-off ' of cœnæsthesia ceases to function, and its unused, abnormally irreducible components adhere to the formations of clear consciousness. In mental disease, the practical activity, both intellectual and social, is altered ; while the purely psychic activity remains unaltered. There is a certain degree of automatism, however, in the patients' behaviour, the residue of their interior participation in our intellectual and social life.

This presupposes another and not less interesting conception, namely, that our normal conscious life is not peculiar to the individual, but to the species to which he belongs. It is socialized consciousness. If the brain is the organ of thought, it is the organ of socialized thought, and not of individual consciousness alone. The brain is the organ of the social psyche. This view of Blondel's can be harmonized with Freud's theories, according to which psychic ill-health consists in conflict between the conscious and the unconscious.

⁴ Karl Jaspers, *Allgemeine Psychopathologie*, etc. (2nd revised edition, Berlin, 1920).

⁵ Ernst Kretschmer, *Der sensitive Beziehungswahn, ein Beitrag zur Paranoiafrage und zur psychiatrischen Charakterlehre* (Berlin, 1918). In his " Gedanken über die Fortentwicklung der psychiatrischen Systematik ", which appeared in the *Zeitsch. f. d. ges. Neurol. u. Psych.*, 48, 1919, and also in " Die psychopathologische Forschung und ihr Verhältnis zur heutigen klin. Psychiatrie ", published ibid., 57, 1920, Kretschmer has abandoned his former rigid dogmatism. See further idem : *Medizinische Psychologie. Ein Leitfaden f. Studium und Praxis* (Leipzig, 1922). [Also Kretschmer's *Physique and Character*, an Investigation of the Theory of Temperament, London, 1925, in the International Library of Psychology, Philosophy, and Scientific Method.]

[6] For the definition of insanity the reader is referred to the various text-books on mental diseases. The reader may also consult S. De Sanctis, *Patologia e Profilassi mentale* (Milan, 1911). The question of normality, abnormality, and insanity may be found summarized in the psychological study of Giacomo Donati, *Le penombre dell' anima* (Ferrara, 1922). Bleuler's conception is also worthy of note : *Lehrbuch der Psychiatrie*, 2nd edition, op. cit. On p. 126 this writer emphatically states : " No limits exist in insanity (Irresein) any more than they exist in other disease." . . . " Many nervous subjects are to-day described as psycho-neuropaths, but by this is intended to be understood those suffering from nervous trouble of psychic origin. The lay mind considers the neurotic as psychically sane, because it is incapable of recognizing the connection between the symptoms and the psyche, either in cause or in effect. The physician must distinguish between cases of psycho-neuroses and of psychoses, *sensu strictiori*, because the delimitation of psychoses, for practical purposes, is made in accordance with social criteria, rather than purely medical standards." Cf. Bleuler, p. 129.

[7] The pathological theory is still maintained by certain writers. At least some psychiatrists and biologists have shown a tendency to equate the emotions arising from religious phenomena with pathological emotions. Cf. Stanley Hall, op. cit., vol. ii, p. 312. The little book of Dr. L. Perrier, *Le sentiment religieux a-t-il une origine pathologique ?* (Paris, 1912), p. 62, may also be read in this connection. A large number of psychologists and psycho-pathologists consider that religious phenomena are derived from suggestion, and in consequence they regard religion as verging towards the pathological. Cf. the recent work of James B. Pratt, *The Religious Consciousness* (New York and London, 1920). This is an interesting book of some 500 pages. On the theory of conversion, the writer's point of view is that of suggestion, determined by a pre-existing theological scheme. The delicate point is to decide the exact significance of suggestion. It is now well known that suggestion is regarded by psychologists as a phenomenon of normal psychology.

[8] Wm. James, op. cit. A masterly application of the conception of ' value ' in religious phenomena has been made by Höffding. Cf. his *Philosophy of Religion*, op. cit., chapter i and elsewhere ; an interesting work on all the psychological questions of religion, containing a good bibliography. The reader's attention is also drawn to other works of this author.

[9] A. Renda, " La teoria psicologica dei valori," which appeared in *Bilychnis*, October and November, 1920.

[10] Giuseppe Portigliotti, *S. Francesco d'Assisi e le epidemie mistiche del medio-evo, studio psichiatrico*, undated. The preface

i s dated from Genoa, 1909. The author maintains the pathological theory.

[11] For a conscientious and authoritative account of Italian mysticism, the reader is referred to E. Gebhart, *L'Italia mistica— Storia del rinascimento religioso del medio evo*, Italian translation by A. Perotti (Bari, 1910). In Chapter III there is an account of St. Francis and of the Franciscan Apostolate. But to understand it thoroughly it is essential to be familiar with the religious and moral conditions of Italy before the time of Joachim of Floris. These are referred to in the first chapter of the work.

[12] Cf. E. Récéjac, *Essai sur les fondements de la connaissance mystique* (Paris, 1897). An excellent book, containing a good discussion of hallucination and the other so-called pathological phenomena of mysticism, cf. pp. 165, 175, 180 et seq. The writer demonstrates that in sane mysticism there are certain subjective phenomena due, not to insanity, but to the imagination. For the question of insanity see Chapter II.

[13] Th. Ribot, *Les maladies de la personnalité* (Paris, 1885).

[14] Havelock Ellis, *The Evolution of Modesty*, op. cit.

[15] References to the religious rites of all ages are to be found in all works on the history of religion and social psychology. Cf. Franz Cumont, *Le Religioni orientali nel paganesimo romano* ; Italian translation by L. Salvatorelli (Bari, 1913). An extremely good book, rich in notes and bibliography, containing accounts and commentaries on the cults of Asia Minor, Egypt, Syria, Persia, as well as astrology and magic. [English translation, *The Oriental Religions in Roman Paganism*, London, 1911.]

[16] Th. Ribot, *Logique des sentiments* (Paris, 1905), op. cit.

[17] A. Forel, *La question sexuelle* (English translation, *The Sexual Question*). (Italian translation by Carlo Rühl, Turin, 1907.) An authoritative work, which deals briefly with all the aspects. There is no suggestion of sensuality, as is usual in almost all books of this description. Particularly interesting is chapter v, on love and the other irradiations of the sexual appetite in the human soul. See also chap. xii, p. 364 et seq., on religion and the sexual life.

At the present time a lively discussion is in progress as to the instinctive bases of religion. There are those who maintain the existence of an original religious instinct in man. Others, again, derive religion from the emotions of admiration and reverence, asserting that admiration is the fusion of the emotions of wonder and of negative self-feeling. The opinion most generally held is that the fundamental emotion of religion is fear. In this connection the reader may consult an article in the *American Journal of Religious Psychology*, vol. ii, by J. H. Leuba : " Fear, Awe, and the Sublime." All works which deal with social psychology are concerned with the psychological origins of religion. Cf. for example, Wm. McDougall, *An Introduction to Social Psychology* (London, 1908, 9th edition, 1915), chap. xiii.

I have no wish to deny the connection between eroticism and religion. The arguments in proof of it are these : the similarity between religious ecstasy and the erotic orgasm (Krafft-Ebing) ; religion is a compensation for disillusions of love ; among the insane, religion and eroticism are not infrequently combined ; in certain of the religions of primitive peoples, the rites are of sexual origin ; cruelty, for instance, is in many religions associated with sensuality ; at the culminating point of their development the passions of religion and sex present a similarity in the quantity and the quality of emotional excitement, and can be substituted the one for the other, when the circumstances are propitious ; and as Krafft-Ebing has pointed out, under pathological influences eroticism and religion are equally liable to be transformed into cruelty.

The criticism of the theory based on the data mentioned above is fully set forth in the text. The affinities between eroticism and religion are not specific ; this is because religion, like art, is also love. The aberrations of erotic mysticism—as I have stated in the text—prove nothing more than the affinity of their origin. In individual cases, exceptional factors can also be admitted. There can, for example, be no doubt that the sexual interrogation, to which certain libertine or incautious confessors subject their penitents, gives rise to aberrations of erotic mysticism, in those individuals whose mental conditions provide a suitable nidus. This opinion is the result of my own medical experience, without reference to the famous revelations of the Canadian Chiniqui, who went over from Catholicism to Protestantism.

[18] Cf. Ivan Bloch, op. cit., p. 78.

[19] A. Kielholz, " Jakob Boehme ; ein pathographischer Beitrag zur Psychologie der Mystik " : *Schriften zur angewandten Seelenkunde*, xvii (Vienna, 1919). In this psycho-analytical study, the author seeks to explain the steps by which Boehme, from being a humble shoemaker, became a mystic theosophist writer. The writer indicates certain phases in the processes of Boehme's pathological mysticism, which do not here concern us. It is certain that sexuality influenced the whole of Boehme's system. This, however, by no means implies that alongside of the pathological phenomena in Boehme there are not also profound matters of considerable cultural importance.

[20] See the remarks on the infamous Rasputin by Portigliotti in the *Quaderni di psichiatria*, Sept. and Oct., 1918.

[21] O. Pfister, " Hysterie und Mystik bei Margare he Ebner (1291-1351) " in the *Zentralblatt für Psychoanalyse*, i, 1910.

[22] Madame Gervaisais, in the novel of the de Goncourt brothers, was a wealthy Parisienne, an intellectual and a free-thinker, whose opinions on religion were derived from Dougald Stewart, Reid, Kant, and Jouffroy. Madame Gervaisais, a widow and mother of a mentally deficient son, was a woman without love, and suffering from tuberculosis. On leaving Paris, she went to live in Papal Rome. There the environment, the sacred music, the visits to churches, the ceremonies of Holy Week, and the suggestion of a fervent Polish Catholic woman, and, further, the violent perorations of a preacher in the Chiesa del Gesù, slowly changed the affects and the ideas of Madame Gervaisais. At first all unconsciously, and then with complacence, she revived her childish religious experience, which at last led to her conversion to Catholicism. She recorded in her diary the inner reasons of her conversion, quoting, at the dawn of day on the feast of St. Agatha, the words of St. Bernard, *Amo Cristum, amo quia amo, amo ut amem.*

Up to this point, the case of Madame Gervaisais presented no morbid features. It is well to emphasize that the two de Goncourts were evidently convinced that conversion is a manifestation of love. The plot of the novel, however, is the story of a sick woman. The formation of her new moral systemization and her new habits demonstrate the irreparable psychic shipwreck of the unfortunate tubercular woman. The psychologist cannot avoid the issue : either *Madame Gervaisais* is a poor artificial novel, or else the authors wished to describe a pathological conversion. In the post-conversional period we find that the fading of her "spiritual sensations" is in no way compensated. The soul of this convert is as arid as a " land parched for want of water ". None of the post-conversional phenomena described by James, and by the present author in chapter vii, are to be met with in the case of Madame Gervaisais. Nothing is evident excepting the signs of cerebral anaemia and exhaustion, which correspond to the course of the progressive pulmonary tuberculosis. The convert not only renounces everything, but in the preoccupation of the purely selfish culture of her soul, grows forgetful of others, and becomes cruel to those around her, and even towards her only son. In fact, in Madame Gervaisais there is a total absence of the " sanctity of life ". It is quite impossible to believe that the de Goncourts were unaware of their heroine's pathological mentality. I quote their words : " In spite of the ardour, the passion of her devotion, the tenacity of her prayers, and her constant concentration on God . . . in spite of all she had done to have God born within her, God was not born . . . She did not possess the Presence. . . . She was afraid of God." (Cf. paragraph xcvii.) In another passage the authors allude to " the apathetic calm which raised her above human emotions " (paragraph lxxvi) and of " the abyss of indifference " into which she had fallen . . . and of her having " become unconscious of even religion itself ", etc., etc. Nor does the end of Madame Gervaisais justify the imaginary process of her conversion. The rapidity with which she returned to reality after her encounter with her brother, and the appearance in her of kindness, which followed after her awakening from her religious stupor, altering her actions and her heart, are nothing but flashes of the soul which belonged to the pre-conversional period of this unhappy woman, who died of hæmoptysis in the ante-chamber of the Pope. (*Madame Gervaisais*, by Edmond and Jules de Goncourt, Paris, 1869.)

[23] In connection with the discussion on the revelations of the devout, I would refer the reader to Henry Joly's *La Psychologie des Saints* (15th edition, Paris, 1912).

[24] Many authors have described the ' visions ' and ' supernatural words ' which are to be met with in the experiences of the mystics. The theologians classify them thus as *corporeal*, *imaginary*, and *intellectual*. In the *corporeal phenomena* there is a real impression. In the *imaginary phenomena* the image is of the briefest duration. In the *intellectual phenomena* there is no sensory representation at all. The Catholic Church is extremely doubtful as to many visions and does not guarantee their authenticity. The Catholic mystics themselves, such as St. Theresa, St. John of the Cross, and St. Ignatius, have declared that such spiritual favours should not be an object of desire, and that they are to be accepted with caution, because they lend themselves so readily to illusion and self-deception.

De Montmorand alludes to these phenomena in chapters v and vi of his work already quoted. The author refers to the interesting views on the subject held by Eugène-Bernard Leroy. See also an article by Mignard, " L'Imagination objectivante et les hallucinations visuelles vraies " in the *Journal de Psychologie Normale et Pathologique* (Paris, 15th June, 1922).

[25] The article, already quoted, on the fiftieth anniversary of Ratisbonne's conversion.

[26] Cf. *L'Abregé des Ouvrages d'Emanuel Swedenborg* (Stockholm, 1788). (Or the English edition of the works of Swedenborg, London, 1891 to 1907.)

[27] H. Delacroix, *Études d'histoire et de psychologie du mysticisme* (Paris, 1908), p. 427 et seq.

[28] The reader should consult the treatise of Baillarger on hallucinations, crowned by the French Academy on 17th December, 1844. Baillarger is referred to in all works on psychiatry I prefer, however, to draw from his original treatise certain of his views which throw light upon my theme. In

paragraph 3, p. 311, the author says that hallucinations of sight are commonly met with among normal persons, and that they represent either the ideas with which the individual has been preoccupied or very vivid sensations he has experienced. On page 369 the author states that psychic hallucinations have been known to the mystics of all ages : " qui sous ce rapport, ont à mon avis, beaucoup mieux compris la nature des hallucinations que les médecins eux-mêmes." On page 383 and page 422, on the subject of psychic hallucinations, the writer concludes that psycho-sensory hallucinations are frequently produced by toxic agencies, while " l'état intellectuel des malades qui ont des hallucinations psychiques diffère peu de celui des personnes qui ont l'habitude de parler seules."

Brierre de Boismont's *Des hallucinations* is a classic on the subject (Paris, 1845, and 1852).

[29] J. Séglas, *Leçons cliniques sur les maladies mentales et nerveuses* (Paris, 1895). Cf. on the subject of hallucinations, the first lecture. There is no need for the reader to make a deep study of the complicated subject of hallucinations, which has been treated with great success in Italy by Tamburini, followed by Tanzi. There are, however, certain questions in regard to voluntary hallucinations which may be found to be of considerable interest to some readers in P. Dheur and J. Moreau's *Les hallucinations volontaires (L'etat hallucinatoire)*, etc. (Paris, 1899). The history of hallucination is given in Chapter III ; voluntary hallucinations are dealt with in Chapter VII.

Those interested in other schools of psychopathology may consult Störring, *Vorlesungen über Psychopathologie* (Leipzig, 1900), 5th chapter, a valuable work with a good bibliography.

[30] On 'the subject of pseudo-hallucination see E. Lugaro's article in the *Rivista di pat. nerv. e ment.*, Jan. and Feb., 1903, on the " Allucinazione psichiche di Baillarger ". See also Tanzi and Lugaro, *Trattato delle malattie mentali* (Milan, 1914), 2nd edition, vol. i, p. 254. [English version, *A Text-book of Mental Diseases*, London, 1909.]

[31] A classification and interpretation of the phenomena of psychic contrast was made some time ago by myself. Cf. Sante De Sanctis, " Psicopatologia delle idee di negazione ", in the *Manicomio moderno* (vol. xvi, No. 3, Nocera Inferiore, 1900). Kräpelin has been deeply occupied by the phenomena of conflict in his treatise, and Bleuler also, op. cit. Among mystics I have never noticed a " psychic clash ", a spirit of contradiction, or ideas of negation, nor have I been able to discover, with any certainty, antagonistic hallucinations.

[32] For the Sienese mystics, and especially Brandano, see Pietro Misciatelli's *Mistici Senesi*, op. cit. This book contains excellent

studies of Filippo degli Agazzari, Bl. Giovanni Colombini, St. Catherine of Siena, St. Bernardino of Siena, and L'Ochino.

[33] On Naundorff see the article of Sérieux and Capgras, " Le messianisme d'un faux Dauphin " in the *Journal de psychol. normale et path.*, 1912.

[34] Giacomo Barzellotti, *Il Monte Amiata e il suo Profeta (David Lazzaretti)* (Milan, 1910).

[35] The subject of constitutions and of constitutional anomalies according to the theories of Viola, Tandler, Bauer, Kraus, Martius, etc., is now well known in Italy owing to Pende's work of popularization. The reader should refer to N. Pende's *Le debolezze di costituzione, Introduzione alla Patologia costituzionale*, Part I, which deals with general theories (Rome, 1922). See particularly chapter i. It must be strongly emphasized that the difficulty in medical practice of distinguishing between a constitutional disease and an anomalous diathesis or constitution, is no excuse for confusing the two conceptions, which should always be kept absolutely distinct.

Ernst Kretschmer, *Physique and Character*, op. cit., has written a most interesting book, which presents the doctrine of constitutions and temperaments, although I am unable to accept all the author's views, and am persuaded that his contribution to modern psychiatry on this subject is less considerable than it appears.

[36] S. De Sanctis, "Studi di Neuro-psichiatria infantile : i fanciulli psicopatici in generale " in the *Archiv. gen. di Neur. e Psich.* (vol. i, No. 1, Naples, 1920). The distinctive classification is here made between the substratum (or the constitution), the orientation (or morbid characteristics), and the *clinical* determination (or disease).

[37] The question of the direct correlation of genius and physical and mental abnormality has long been profoundly studied ; most recently in Italy by Patrizi. His studies of Leopardi and Caravaggio are well known.

[38] The number of epileptics with what is termed an *intellectual aura*, is small. Nevertheless, in my own long practice I have met with more than one case, and I took at the time a special note of the ideas and representations forming the aura. Actually in none of my cases did I find a concept of any value, although several of my patients were persons of high intelligence. As a rule, when it was not a matter of simple phrases or a musical motif, they were ordinary ideas, trite statements, proverbs, and most frequently memories of things read or learnt long ago. I do not wish to attach too much importance to this, but the reader will perhaps agree that it is of some significance for the argument in the text.

[39] It cannot be denied that in certain individual cases it is extraordinarily difficult to make a clear differential diagnosis between the mystics who are *chronically insane* and the mystics whom we have called *exceptional* (saints, prophets, or heroes). Unless we are willing to base the entire difference on a pragmatic standard—which is what the scientist should endeavour as far as possible to avoid—it is essential to look for certain differential symptoms. Therefore it cannot be too often repeated that those mystics who are chronic dements, even those who frequently win popular favour, can in my opinion be distinguished from exceptional persons by the following analytical tests : 1, by their thoughts, and still more by their actions, both of which markedly contradict common experience and logic ; reality, even when recognized, is not elaborated and experienced in accordance with this recognition ; 2, the subject does not follow tradition, but is always an innovator ; 3, with the lapse of years, the subject's mentality deteriorates in thought and action ; 4, innovator or not, the chronically insane mystic consciously or unconsciously follows a selfish path, or one which satisfies his own ordinary desires.

Reformers and innovators, when chronically insane, are invariably on a low ethical level. This is a criterion undoubtedly of real value. From the psycho-pathological aspect, therefore, their immorality signifies this : the mental disease has set up such an obstacle in consciousness, that the ancient or pre-social subconscious which has been set free cannot undergo sufficient elaboration for social purposes. But when, in spite of the obstacle imposed by the mental disease, there is no apparent sign of immorality—which does happen, though rarely, in paranoiac subjects—this can only be accounted for by one of two reasons : either the ' pre-social' subconscious mind is not liberated integrally, on account of ' obstacles ' or inhibitions, belonging to the subconscious sphere itself ; or because a more or less ' recent ' subconscious is liberated, which already bears the marks of morality. In such circumstances, which, however, are very rare, the case would present serious difficulties in diagnosis.

CHAPTER VIII

[1] We have already dealt with psychic systems and complexes. It will suffice here merely to add that, to-day, there exists a technique by means of which it is possible to provoke the reappearance at the higher levels of consciousness, of the more deeply sunken psychic systems. It is profoundly important in psychopathology and in legal and criminal psychology as well as in everyday life and in pedagogy, that we be able

to avail ourselves of what may be termed the *semeiotic of the subconscious*, that is, a series of *Komplexmerkmale*.

We are now able to recall complexes by psycho-physiological means, through the method of association, and by various other psycho-analytical methods. The reader may consult on this matter Samuel C. Kohs: "The Association Method in its Relation to the Complex and Complex Indicators," in the *American Journal of Psychology* (October, 1914). This is an exhaustive study with an excellent bibliography.

² Almost all religions possess associations, committees, periodicals, etc., devoted to propaganda. It is scarcely necessary to mention the famous Congregation *De propaganda fide*, besides which there are the well-known Catholic missions, as well as Protestant missionary societies and institutions. A remarkable institution exists for this purpose in Germany at the present time, the *Winfried-Bund*, which controls the organized efforts directed towards the conversion of Protestants to Catholicism in Germany. On the occasion of the Second General Congress of the *Bund*, which was held in 1921, at Paderborn, the objects of the League were clearly defined as: 1, the revival of the true faith among the Catholic population; 2, work among Protestants; 3, the tutelage of converts. See the report of the Second General Meeting of the Winfried-Bund held 25th August, 1921, at Paderborn (published by the Bonifacius Drückerei, Paderborn). Propaganda connected with all the various religions is systematically and efficiently organized. For instance, at the conference of the above-mentioned League, Father Gisbert Menge advocated, as a means of propaganda, the holding of meetings, where an address, or lecture, on Catholic truth, should be followed by recitations and music of a high order. The powerful attraction of Dante for non-Catholics, was emphasized by the Landesrat von Tiedemann as a possible source of conversion; Bishop Hähling recommended the positive explanation of the truths of Christianity and the avoidance of polemical and controversial discussion. Frau von Tiedemann, who had herself become a convert through the reading of Kunz's book (*Der Heilige Franz von Assisi*, Munich, 1908), advocated that conversions be followed by religious instruction to converts who had recently entered the Church.

The Protestant propaganda throughout Italy, as every observer knows, is extremely active, especially in the south. The daily press has described the Anglican propaganda which is being extensively undertaken by the English in Russia, and so forth.

INDEX TO PROPER NAMES